Drugs and the Aged

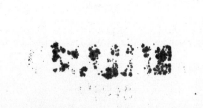

Drugs and the Aged

William D. Poe, M.D., F.A.C.P.

Chief, Intermediate (Geriatric) Medicine
Veterans Administration Medical Center
Salem, Virginia
Associate Professor of Medicine
University of Virginia Medical School
Charlottesville, Virginia

Donald A. Holloway, B.S., Phar. D.

Pharmacist, Methodist Retirement Homes
Durham, North Carolina
Pharmacist, Duke University Hospital
Durham, North Carolina

McGraw-Hill Book Company

New York St. Louis San Francisco Auckland Bogotá Düsseldorf
Johannesburg London Madrid Mexico Montreal New Delhi Panama
Paris São Paulo Singapore Sydney Tokyo Toronto

DRUGS AND THE AGED

Copyright © 1980 by McGraw-Hill, Inc. All rights reserved. Printed in the United States of America. No part of this publication may be reproduced, stored in a retrieval system, or transmitted, in any form or by any means, electronic, mechanical, photocopying, recording, or otherwise, without the prior written permission of the publisher.

1234567890 DODO 7832109

This book was set in Times Roman by Allyn-Mason, Incorporated. The editors were Richard S. Laufer and Irene Curran; the cover was designed by Tana Klugherz; the production supervisor was Milton J. Heiberg.
R. R. Donnelley & Sons Company was printer and binder.

Library of Congress Cataloging in Publication Data

Poe, William D   date
    Drugs and the aged.

    Includes bibliographical references and index.
    1. Geriatric pharmacology. 2. Drugs and the aged.
I. Holloway, Donald A., joint author. II. Title.
RC953.7.P63   618.9′7′06   79-15451
ISBN 0-07-050330-3

Contents

Preface

From 1970 to 1975 we, the authors, found ourselves in a pleasant working relationship. We enjoyed a fortuitous meeting of minds regarding the use of drugs in old people. The potential for harm in any prescription, the need for economy in the use of drugs where money is limited, a growing realization of the frequent misuses of drugs in patients coming under our care, the importance of the manner and attitude of nurses who administered drugs, the legitimate use of placebos, an awareness of subtle signs of drug intoxication or overdose — all indicated to us that pharmacy in the aged had not received enough attention, that it had, indeed, become something of a specialty.

This book, then, is a logical extension of our experience and study in a natural laboratory, the Methodist Retirement Homes in Durham, North Carolina. The number of old people there is around 200. While we worked together, very few residents had other personal physicians and fewer still purchased drugs elsewhere. A natural communication developed between us that we believe others should share: physicians, pharmacists, students, social workers, nurses, therapists, administrators, and yes, patients and their families.

Where there is more than one author, a book may have an unevenness of style. We have tried to overcome this by fully editing each other. For example, a sentence from each of us may occur in the same paragraph. On the other hand, there has been a division of labor. Dr. Holloway, by and large, is responsible for much of the organization, the gathering of data, and the proper citation of references. Dr. Poe has written from his experience as a geriatrician, author, and medical teacher.

We hope we have put together a useful book of lasting benefit to those who use it.

William D. Poe
Donald A. Holloway

Drugs and the Aged

Chapter 1

Introduction

Since World War II, especially in the sixties and seventies, a number of forces have come together to claim the attention of society at large. Among the more important are: (1) more people are living longer and as they do, they require more medicine; and (2) the proportion of the very old among the elderly is steadily increasing (see Figure 1-1). These are the facts which will concern us throughout this book.

Professor Leonard Hayflick of Stanford University has written extensively on population and longevity. He states that

> ...if zero population growth can be achieved, it can be predicted that by 2025 A.D. those over 65 will number nearly 40 million and will constitute more than 20 percent of the total population...
>
> The inevitable consequence would be a further acceleration of current trends in which the government would be providing more health care, food, housing, recreation, and income to the elderly. Since it could safely be assumed that the proportion of those in government over 65 would also increase, the closest thing to a gerontocracy could prevail in 2025.[1]

What Hayflick is saying is what those of us who have been in geriatrics or gerontology have realized for years. We believe that housing, health care, phar-

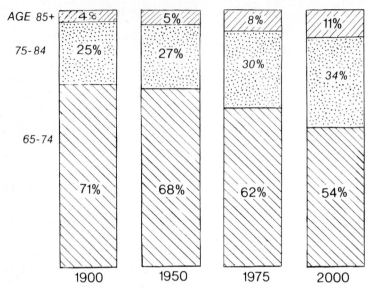

AGE 85+ 4%

75-84 25%

65-74

71%

1900

5%

27%

68%

1950

8%

30%

62%

1975

11%

34%

54%

2000

Figure 1-1   The proportion of the very old among the elderly is increasing. *(The National Center for Health Statistics.)*

macy, social services, government, business, education, nutrition, religion, construction, and manufacturing, i.e., nearly the entire national enterprise, must be directed toward the changing age of the nation's citizens. Furthermore, old people will have the political power to bring about the changes that an older society demands.

Some would view a gerontocracy with loathing, or at least with tolerant condescension. On the other hand, such a society might be called upon to balance the excesses and degeneracy that have pervaded much of American life in the past 25 years.

Certainly, one wholesome effect of large numbers of old people would be that they could help themselves and their contemporaries to regain the self-respect that was lost in a harsh, youth-oriented society. Maybe old people could learn to stand on their own merits rather than pretend—with cosmetic surgery, wigs, and dyed hair—to be something they are not.

There are now about 20 million people over 65 in the United States. There are area agencies on aging in about 600 communities. There is an Administration on Aging in the Department of Health, Education, and Welfare. In 1975, a National Institute on Aging was established in the National Institutes of Health to be concerned with basic research on aging and its problems. The U. S. Department of Agriculture has a program to enhance the nutrition of old people.

Many universities, ever alert to justify their existence, are starting training programs in gerontology, the study of aging in its broader aspects. One proposal suggests that 1000 Ph.D.s a year be trained to deal with aging—enough, in 5 years, to put 100 of them in every state, and, in 10 years, to put one in all but the smallest town. Thus, the prospect of a neighborhood gerontologist is not as farfetched as it may at first sound.

The social work profession, always sensitive to human need, has probably led in the awareness of the sheer massiveness of the problems presented by many old people—health, housing, income, transportation, family relationships, and nutrition. More social workers will undoubtedly become involved with elderly people as the numbers of each increase.

Many religious and fraternal organizations are taking literally the psalmist's injunction: "Cast me not off in the time of old age; forsake me not when my strength faileth" (Psalms 71:9). Retirement villages, nursing homes, day-care centers, and special programs are in various stages of development under the auspices of nearly every denomination. Where there were ministers to youth, in many places there are now ministers to the aged as well. As in many endeavors, Jewish agencies often have led in providing homes, hospitals, services, and facilities for the elderly.

In large measure a result of political forces, physicians, nurses, hospitals, and schools for health professionals are paying greater attention to the problems of old people. There are several fully developed programs for special training in geriatrics or geriatric medicine, an emerging specialty. Professional people who have special experience with the elderly are receiving increasing respect in hospitals, schools, and universities. For example, there are chairs of geriatric medicine in at least five or six medical schools, whereas only one existed 3 years ago. The Veterans Administration recently appointed an assistant chief for extended care and is emphasizing chronic illness, which affects mostly elderly people. It appears that geriatrics will soon be a fully developed specialty, a specialty that will require the abilities of many allied health workers, social workers, nurses, psychologists, therapists, and others.

As a result of the widespread concern about aging, it is clear that many people need to be aware of what may be going on chemically and pharmacologically in the bodies of old people. Such knowledge should not be confined to physicians and pharmacists. The problems of drug management should claim the attention of any well-informed person who deals with old people, especially someone in one of the helping professions. Where there is knowledge of drug management it needs emphasis; not a day passes in an active geriatrics practice when there is not a patient seen with symptoms and signs of drug misuse.

Someone estimated that old people, roughly 10 percent of the population, consume about 25 percent of the medicine sold in the United States. When one considers that medicine manufacturing is measured in billions of dollars in the United States, to say nothing of huge international companies around the world producing medicines, one can get some idea about how much medicine old people consume. If at one time, 20 million people take an average of four prescription drugs, the total amount of medicine taken is enormous, leading, potentially, to an enormous amont of misery.

Is all this medicine necessary, or even desirable? Certainly it is not. Human nature being what it is, though, medicine consumption and overconsumption is understandable. Greek gods and goddesses sought potions that would do wondrous things for their friends or fiendish things to their foes. Medicine shows of a past generation promised youth, vitality, and beauty. Television of the present day makes it appear abnormal if all of us are not taking something for digestion, arthritis, fungal infections, or bowel "regularity." Many people are seduced into believing that a hard day or a poor night's sleep cannot happen to a person unless there is something wrong, to be righted by pill or potion.

With lifelong tendencies to seek bliss or beauty from a bottle, it is little wonder that old people, with their problems, often resort to what has been called "multipharmacy" or "polypharmacy," i.e., the taking of many medicines.

We are convinced that *the overuse, misuse, or abuse of drugs is a major and frequent cause of illness in old people*. We shall try to document this conclusion as we go along. Certainly, we are in distinguished company, whose views we share. Doctor Oliver Wendell Holmes, well known as a poet but a distinguished physician as well, inveighed against overprescribing by his fellow physicians. Sir William Osler lectured against the use of too many medicines. George Bernard Shaw good-naturedly castigated the medical profession in the introduction to *The Doctor's Dilemma* for prescribing too much too often. In the present generation, a number of leading physicians have stated, in effect, that drugs are dangerous and occasionally deadly. Nevertheless, drug use continues to increase year by year.

Newspapers carry story after story of scandal in prescribing and in dispensing drugs. Fraud is frequently cited as a dollars-and-cents issue. Maybe there is negligence in not recognizing the harm medicines can do.

Data indicates an unfavorable reaction in 1 patient out of 9 on a hospital medical service, where drugs are prescribed and given by professional people. It is horrible to consider the number of mistakes old people can make if they are forgetful, cannot read directions clearly, misunderstand, or are governed entirely by their feelings of the moment. No person can easily keep up with more than three of four prescriptions, yet it is not at all unusual for some old people to be taking 15 or 20 different medicines.

How can this be? Too much medicine results from its easy availability and a lack of awareness of its harm, in addition to the human tendency to take something for what ails you. It is far easier for a physician to innocently prescribe a drug for dizziness, say, than to probe and question about all the medicines an old person is taking. Mr. K., an elderly man obviously not serously ill, wanted something for his swimming head. Only after a prolonged conversation did it become evident that he was half drunk part of the time—definitely something to be hidden in the fundamentalist community in which he lived. It is far easier for a physician to prescribe than to think. It is far easier for a family to demand medication for an old relative than it is to give love and acceptance. It is far easier for a nurse to pop a pill in someone's old mouth than to give a back rub. It is far easier to "do something" than to give one's self. Philosophically, this last probably is at the root of the problems of our society, especially the drug problems that come to the surface in old age.

In the following chapter we shall explain something about the metabolism of drugs. In doing so, we will appeal to the general reader. To those who wish to explore more deeply the chemical reactions of drugs, we refer to standard works on biochemistry and pharmacology. We will discuss common symptoms of drug intolerance or intoxication. Several chapters will be devoted to various classes of drugs such as laxatives and tranquilizers. Finally, we shall relate our views and experience about proprietary versus generic drugs, the cost of drugs, the use of placebos, and the interactions among various health professionals.

REFERENCES

1 Leonard Hayflick, "2025 A.D.: Aging in America's Future," *Proceedings of a Symposium in Dedication of the Pharmaceutical Research Center and Medical Administration Building,* Hoechst-Roussel Pharmaceuticals, Inc., Somerville, N.J., Nov. 7, 1975, p.31.

Chapter 2

Metabolism and Pharmacokinetics

Metabolism is the sum total of life's chemical and physical processes. It is what happens to the food we eat and the water we drink. It is what becomes of all of us as we become ill or get old. It goes on as long as life lasts and stops only when we die. It explains the differences between young and old, big and little, slow and fast, smart and stupid. Of course, not all these differences are fully understood, and metabolism does not always decide a person's fate. Goodness and evil, environment, and experience are all important in what a person is or becomes; but metabolism may determine one's potential.

Let us take a simple example. How does a plant grow? The simplest plant lives on a simple sugar. Through the action of light, carbon dioxide in the atomosphere and water in the air or in the soil are combined to manufacture enough glucose, a simple sugar, for the plant to grow and reproduce. As it does so it gives off oxygen, important in the metabolism of higher animals, including humans.

Human beings live basically on three kinds of foodstuffs—fats, proteins, and carbohydrates. These can be extremely complex chemical compounds, but basically we live on the same things as plants and other animals. Thus, we nourish ourselves by ingestion of plants and other animals composed chiefly of carbon, nitrogen, hydrogen, and oxygen. Metabolism, then, is the digestion, absorption, transport, utilization, chemical change, and excretion of foodstuffs, and the changes in the body necessary to accomplish these processes.

When applied to drugs, however, metabolism takes on a different meaning. The reason for this is not simply a fondness for big words such as *pharmacokinetics* and *pharmacodynamics*. Drugs are not food. They are foreign substances. Though they frequently do good, they are, almost by definition, capable of doing harm. Because they are foreign substances they have no place in the proper functioning of the metabolism of a healthy person. Drugs, then, may be defined as foreign substances which through their action, physical or chemical, influence the living organism. As prescribed by physicians, drugs are foreign substances to be ingested, injected, inhaled, applied, or rubbed on to produce a pharmacological effect, that is, to produce a specific drug action.

Types of Drug Effects

Let's start with a simple example. When procaine or one of its chemical relatives is applied to the mucus-secreting surfaces of the mouth or nose, it reacts chemically to render the nerve endings insensitve to pain. When injected locally, these *local anesthetics* relieve pain caused by injury or stimulation of sensitive nerve endings. From one point of view, this is about as simple an example of drug action as we know. Yet, the exact chemical reactions involving pain and its prevention are in general not known, in spite of a great deal of research.

Now let's be a bit more sophisticated. If aspirin is to be used for muscle soreness it is swallowed. It is then absorbed from the upper small intestine into the bloodstream. It is then pumped to the brain and to the sore muscle. In a way not well understood, it relieves the soreness and acts upon the pain center in the brain to relieve the pain. After a while, it is excreted by the kidneys into the urine.

Other medications may be stored in fatty or connective tissues, the liver, the nervous system, the thyroid gland, or elsewhere. Some may be changed in the liver and excreted in the bile through the gastrointestinal tract with bowel movements. Other medicines may be altered first and then excreted very slowly. *Pharmacokinetics*, then, concerns itself with how much, how long, when, how, if, and where a drug will be absorbed, transported, used, changed, and excreted. To quote Goodman and Gilman, ''Pharmacokinetics deals with the absorption, distribution, biotransformation, and excretion of drugs.''[1]

In a nontechnical sense, one may speak of *''drug metabolism.''* In a narrower sense, such a term is a misnomer and *pharmacokinetics* is then the correct term, which, along with *pharmacodynamics*, consists of ''the study of the biochemical and physiological effects of drugs and their mechanisms of action.''[2] Again, metabolism deals with natural processes. Pharmacokinetics and pharmacodynamics deal with drugs, which are foreign substances.

We may have belabored the point here but a great deal more is known about drug actions than is understood. It is a very broad subject involving chemistry, physics, biology, physiology, and anatomy. Each part of the living organism has its own reaction, each person reacts slightly differently, and much is not known. This is why foreign substances in people should be used with caution. One often cannot predict what effect a given drug will have in a given person. The important questions in administering drugs are not always given due consideration.

Effects of Age

The problems are compounded in old people, and this fact is not fully appreciated either. We shall try to explain why drug reactions are a special problem in old people, and why they tend to be more frequent and more severe. Comfort recently pointed out:

> Older patients today account for about 25 percent of prescriptions, and a higher proportion of office case load, and their numbers are growing. Their symptoms, diagnostics, and reaction to therapies differ as sharply as those of babies from the adult norm as taught: ...they are extremely susceptible to overmedication and mismedication with substances and doses fully appropriate to younger persons. Their problems with the irrational attitudes of society, which treats them as suddenly nonpeople or different people, are apt to be diagnosed as a Valium deficiency[2]

Returning to pharmacokinetics and aging, much is known but hard to measure. It is appropriate to point out well-known differences in older people. An experienced pathologist, a physician who examines tissues through a microscope, can estimate the age of a person. Let us consider some of the cellular changes as one gets older.

The skin becomes thinner and less elastic. The lining of the digestive system, concerned with digestion and absorption, becomes less cellular. Acid and mucus-secreting cells in the stomach become less numerous. Lymphoid cells in the gut become fewer in number. Liver and pancreatic enzymes are secreted in smaller quantities as one gets older. The transport time from mouth to anus may be increased, decreased, or sensitized by age, food, fluid, or medication.

The nervous system controls movement and senses. The automatic movements of the heart, blood vessels, digestive, excretory, respiratory, and reproductive systems are altered. The number of cells in the brain, spinal cord, and ganglia slowly diminishes from about the age of 35.

Nephrons, the excreting units in the kidneys, gradually shrivel and are replaced by scar tissue. Their number is about half as great in an 85-year-old person as in a 25-year-old. Most drugs cannot be excreted as rapidly and tend to accumulate to toxic levels in old people.

The heart does not pump as efficiently in a 40-year-old as in a 20-year-old, nor in an 80-year-old as in a 40-year-old. In technical terms, the afterload—the amount of blood remaining in the ventricle after the heart beats—is greater in the old than in the young. The concept of the failing heart may be in error. There is doubt that the aging heart needs the vigorous treatment often prescribed for the symptoms of heart failure. Geriatricians have often seen that many old people may be made worse by conventional treatment of heart disorders. Even many cardiologists do not fully appreciate the differences that are present in old people.

Alterations of consciousness and perception occur in many old people. There is a normal loss of hearing in old people; they may not hear instructions about the taking of medicines. Some people cannot see to read directions, or to get the right pill, or to measure insulin for injection. A surprising number of people have been conditioned through life to take something for every symptom. When old people are left alone, they tend, like the rest of us, to become introspective and to dwell on symptoms. They are in greater need of diversion than of medicine. We have been amazed, amused, and horrified at the way some people literally orchestrate medicines as a conductor leads an orchestra, calling now for this and then for that instrument or medicament.

Sensations of hunger and thirst are frequently diminished in the elderly. Dehydration, a marked deficiency of fluid, causes weakness and stupor with relative frequency. In the United States, vitamin deficiencies are rare except among old people who are more prone than others to have an inadequate diet. Such inadequacies of food and fluid affect the digestion, absorption, transport, utilization, and excretion of many drugs.

SUMMARY

We have pointed out that drugs may act differently in elderly patients because of changes of structure and of function. In addition, disease states also affect structure and function. Where advanced age, disease, and one drug are present in the same patient there is a strong potential for toxicity. Where age, two or more diseases, and two or more drugs interact, it is more likely than not that there will be an unpleasant or dangerous drug reaction. Of course, as the number of drugs and diseases increases, the chance of a reaction increases proportionately.

In the following chapter we will see how this interaction of patient, drugs, and diseases can take place.

REFERENCES

1   L.S. Goodman and A. Gilman (eds.), *The Pharmacological Basis of Therapeutics,* 5th ed., Macmillan, New York, 1975, p. 1.
2   Alex Comfort, "Geriatrics: A British View" *N. Engl. J. Med.,* **297**:624 (1977).

Chapter 3

The Case of Mrs. O.

THE CASE HISTORY

The following report was taken from among the many cases of drug misuse in the authors' files. It tends to summarize the problems of drug use in the elderly.

Mrs. O., 87, came under our care on May 5, 1977. Over a period of about a year, she had lost her appetite almost completely, 50 pounds in weight, and her desire to live. In effect, she was sent to our institution to live out her few remaining weeks.

She had been in a hospital for almost six weeks, from February to April, and had been tested exhaustively. A stomach x-ray and a bowel x-ray indicated no trouble. Liver and bone scans indicated no evidence of cancer. Exhaustive tests on blood and urine indicated mild anemia and mild kidney failure, not infrequent in many old people. A chest x-ray and repeated electrocardiograms indicated only changes that were not remarkable for a person of such advanced age, mild enlargement of the heart, and a pulse rate of 90.

Special diets and special urging had been tried to get the patient to eat. Food was repulsive to her and she could not eat. If she did, she immediately became nauseated.

In the remote past, some 40 years before her admission, a thyroid deficiency had been diagnosed. Her body had become accustomed to three times the average dose of medication for thyroid deficiency. The dose had even continued through the years. Iron had been prescribed in the hospital for her anemia.

At about the age of 80, she had been given a standard dose of a digitalis preparation for her failing heart, manifested by moderate shortness of breath and slight swelling of her ankles after prolonged sitting. Since leaving the hospital she has had mild diarrhea.

The physical examination revealed a tired, thin, pale, depressed, discouraged elderly women who said she did not want to live. She weighed 94 pounds and could hardly walk unassisted. Her pulse was 100 beats per minute. There were full blood vessels in the neck. The liver was enlarged. The skin was loose, warm, and silky-dry.

It was obvious that this patient was dying of drug intoxication. After another stay in the hospital she was restored to nearly perfect health, not by medication but by omitting it.

Let's see if we can reconstruct what occurred in this now charming, alert, very old woman. It may call for a bit of intuition, since one cannot document exactly what happened in her long medical history. The purpose of this treatise, though, is to improve the intuition of people who work with the elderly when it comes to drug problems.

Intuitively, one might infer that Mrs. O. was tired and depressed in her late forties. Forty years ago, the measurement of thyroid deficiency lacked precision. Many menopausal women were given thyroid because no other hormone was available then. It seemed to help some women, but whether through its pharmacological action or placebo effect no one could be sure. There was an exotic ceremony of having a basal metabolism test in which a tired, middle-aged woman breathed from a measured cylinder of oxygen for a measured length of time. The basal metabolic rate (BMR) was a crude test, but it was complicated, expensive, and awesome enough to be fashionable among intelligent women going through the change of life. Then, too, the test gave a crude, indirect appraisal of thyroid function—a very poor test indeed, but the best of the day. If the doctor were willing, if the patient were susceptible, if the machine didn't leak, if Mrs. O. had had a good night's sleep and had not eaten before the test, and if she were not nervous when her nose was clamped and a mask put over her mouth, the test might have indicated a thyroid deficiency. Presumably Mrs. O. underwent such a crude test and this is the beginning of our case analysis. At any rate, necessary or not, Mrs. O. got a prescription for thyroid extract, 1 grain (65 milligrams) a day—cheap, readily available, and relatively harmless. In addition, she got a diagnosis that was difficult to escape from. Thyroid medication virtually nullified the value of subsequent tests of thyroid function.

With life's vicissitudes, the waxing and waning of euphoria and depression, the dose was gradually increased to 3 grains a day, not unusual but still a hefty dose. Here the dose had remained until she entered the hospital in February 1977.

About 1970, though, at the age of 80, Mrs. O. developed shortness of breath, fatigue, and mild puffiness of her ankles. This vital, active, alert woman no longer could go up and down the stairs without exhaustion. She could no longer catch the bus and go to the shopping center. Sometimes, she had to prop herself up at night to get her breath. All these symptoms indicated a failing heart, fairly common in old people.

Right here, her physician should have taken stock. Was the thyroid, which speeds metabolism, causing part of the burden on her aging heart? Evidently the question was never asked. Mrs. O., having taken thyroid for nearly 40 years, may not even have told her physician. It was not really a medicine, it was replacement therapy, just something she took every day, like food and drink. Maybe her doctor didn't ask; but if he had asked "Are you taking any medicine?" she probably would have answered "No."

What is the treatment for Mrs. O's failing heart? Ah! Digitalis and a diuretic. Now digitalis, which will be discussed later at length, is an extremely useful drug that comes in several pill sizes. A diuretic helps the body rid itself of water and salt retained in the body when the heart is weak. So a heart overburdened by thyroid was treated not by discontinuing an offending medicine, but by taking two new medicines that can do mischief of their own!

Mrs. O. was started on daily doses of 0.25 milligrams of Lanoxin (a digitalis-type drug) and 40 milligrams of Lasix (a commonly used diuretic). These are standard doses. Slowly, inexorably, the medicine did its work. For a year or so, Mrs. O. did better. At least she was not short of breath. She lost her sparkling vitality, but so do most people at 80 plus. Somehow, she could not eat. Food simply had no appeal. Since she lived alone and was much weaker now, there was no one to go to the shopping center for groceries. She became depressed—not unusual for elderly people living alone. Her son, who lived in a nearby town, came each week. Clearly, his mother was too old to go on. Something needed to be done. The doctor, not fully aware of the use and abuse of drugs in old people, prescribed medicine for depression but, fortunately, stopped it when it did no good. Mrs. O. became alarmingly ill in early 1977 and was put in a nursing home. When she failed to improve and continued to lose weight, she was put in the hospital to see if she had cancer. And this brings our story up to date, out of conjecture into documented fact.

ANALYSIS OF THE CASE

What happened? Thyroid was unnecessary. It increased the burden on an aging heart. It never should have have been prescribed. Once prescribed, it never should have been increased. Old people are particularly sensitive to thyroid medications since they are not as able as young people to store or excrete thyroid hormone. One treatment for a failing heart is to give medicine that suppresses thyroid function. Any time heart failure is treated, thyroid function and medication should be considered. This was the first error.

Digitalis and its chemical cousins can be life-saving, but 80-year-old kidneys exrete it extremely slowly. If a standard dose is given to an old person, it will almost invariably cause a loss of appetite, irregular heart action, nausea, vomiting, diarrhea, disturbed vision, or a worsening of the heart condition. It is difficult to describe the aversion to food digitalis can cause, but more about this later. Lanoxin should not have been prescribed in the standard dose, and this was the second error.

The third error involved the use of a diuretic. Lasix can be life-saving, but it depletes the body of water and salt. With water depletion, blood volume is diminished and many old people already have this problem without the use of medicines. They simply don't feel thirsty. The kidneys cannot excrete waste and drugs unless there is sufficient body water to allow a large flow of urine. Because of the loss of nephrons, (excretory units), old people need more water, not less.

Tests in our hospital showed that Mrs. O. had dehydration and an excess of waste materials and Lanoxin in her blood. The treatment was to discontinue her thyroid, Lanoxin, and Lasix. Incidentally, her anemia was due to poor food intake, and her mild diarrhea cleared spontaneously when the iron she was taking for anemia was discontinued. It may be better to be deprived of medical care than to have medicine prescribed unwisely.

CONCLUSION

Mrs. O. is now a sparkling, active, alert, intelligent woman. In September 1977, she weighed 120 pounds. She demonstrates what we want to get across: *Improperly used medicines are a hazard to your health, especially if you are old.*

In writing about Mrs. O., we have touched on only several symptoms of drug misuse. Now, before considering symptoms at greater length, let's see how drugs work.

Chapter 4

How Drugs Work

It is not our purpose to go deeply into physiology, pharmacology, biochemistry, and anatomy. We are writing for a general audience of educated people. We shall leave the world of radioimmunoassay, fluorescent antibody, and minced mouse brains to laboratory scientists who have a language all their own. To impart a general knowledge of how drugs work, though, does require some basic technical knowledge.

In this chapter we shall give a number of definitions. We shall follow a pill through the body. We shall then explain certain differences between the ways old and young bodies may react to drugs. We believe careful study of this chapter may make the rest of what we have to say relatively easy to understand.

TYPES OF DRUG ACTIONS

Drugs work basically in the following ways;

1 Drugs block nerve impulses. More drugs work in this way than in any other. Returning to procaine, it blocks pain impulses at nerve endings in the mucous membranes. In addition, if injected about the spinal cord, procaine (or one of its chemical relatives) can block the passage of pain impulses to the brain. We'll talk more, much more, about blocking agents.

2 Drugs, in effect, stimulate nerve impulses. Caffeine in coffee is a stimulant. Nicotine in cigarettes is a stimulant.

When a nerve impulse, measured in thousandths of a second, is transmitted to the next nerve it must first cross a gap (synapse) between the two. Near the end of the first nerve are granules which store a neurotransmitter. The impulse causes the granules to release their neurotransmitter into the gap, and the impulse passes over the gap and continues to the next nerve. To prevent constant stimulation of the second nerve, the neurotransmitter must be removed from the gap. Some is resorbed into the first nerve and reenters the storage granules. The remainder is destroyed by enzymes in the nerve cell and gap. At this gap, stimulants and antidepressants act to increase nerve transmission and anesthetics and tranquilizers can decrease it. Stimulants, for example, can increase nervous or physical activity by: (1) inhibiting the destroying enzymes or (2) blocking the resorption of the neurotransmitter into the nerve or the storage granules. Among a dozen or so neurotransmitters are norepinephrine, epinephrine, and serotonin. All are resorbed; all are inactivated chemically by the enzyme monoamine oxidase. Norepinephrine and serotonin are also inactivated by the enzyme catechol-o-methyl transferase. The functions and locations of the neurotransmitters in the brain vary, and drugs affecting them may affect only one or two of them. As a general rule, we can say that stimulants simply remove the "brakes" on physiological functions.

3 Drugs work directly on living cells. Many anticancer drugs work in this way. Antibiotics work directly on living bacterial cells. Ether anesthesia works directly on cells in the higher brain centers to produce its effect.

4 Drugs may work by replacing body deficiencies, e.g., insulin in diabetes and female hormones in women who have absent or diminished ovarian function.

5 Any combination of 1 through 4. This is why many untoward drug reactions occur. A drug may do its job very well indeed by working one way but be near fatal by working in another. For an example, let us return to the case of Mrs. O, who was placed on a digitalis preparation. Digitalis increases the efficiency of heart muscle cells and can be life-saving. However, in Mrs. O.'s case, the digitalis stimulated the vomit center in the brain to the point that she nearly starved to death.

Our readers will have come across such terms as autonomic, sympathetic, parasympathetic, and central nervous system. These terms are useful in medical parlance but can be simplified for the nonmedical reader. Autonomic (look in any dictionary) simply means acting independently of volition, i.e., involuntarily. One does not tell the stomach to pour out its juices after one has swallowed a piece of steak. It is done involuntarily. Life would be terribly complicated if we purposely had to turn on all the switches and pull all the plugs of our existence. God took care of these arrangements by giving us an autonomic (involuntary) nervous system.

This involuntary or autonomic nervous system is composed of two parts: (1) the *sympathetic* system, which is "the part of the autonomic nervous system that contains adrenergic fibers and tends to depress secretion, decrease the tone and contractility of smooth muscle, and cause the contraction of blood vessels," and (2) the *parasympathetic* system, which is "the part of the autonomic nervous system that contains chiefly cholinergic fibers and tends to induce secretion, increase the tone and contractility of smooth muscle, and cause the dilation of blood vessels and that consists of a cranial and sacral part." Yes! Now let's make sense of technical definitions.

Why do many public speakers have a glass of water beside the lectern? Anyone who has ever been severely frightened knows that such a state causes an exceedingly dry mouth. When embarrassed, a susceptible person may get his or her tongue twisted or gulp because the salivary juices just aren't flowing. At the same time there may be an inability to relish food, the pulse may pound, and the person may feel faint. The same phenomena may occur with stage fright, a classic example of sympathetic (adrenergic) autonomic nerve stimulation. The blood vessels contract and the performer pales; the mouth becomes dry; the secretions (see definition) are depressed. The contractility of smooth muscle is reduced. Under stress, a person may have an unusual urge to urinate or defecate. Most of us can understand about sympathetic nerve stimulation. Coffee is a mild stimulant, producing in a minor way some of the symptoms of alertness and fear. Adrenergic stimulation is similar in effect to an injection of adrenalin, a naturally occurring chemical produced by the adrenal glands.

In ascending order of their strength, caffeine, nicotine, ephedrine, amphetamines, and adrenalin produce adrenergic effects. They dry secretions, heighten awareness, raise blood pressure, suppress appetite, and relax smooth muscle. Some of these drugs used to be prescribed frequently but their use has fallen into deserved ill repute. They are used in cold remedies to dry up excessive nasal secretions. *Adrenergic* (adrenaline-like in action) or *sympathomimetic* (sympathetic-like in action) are terms used to describe these drug effects.

Parasympathetic stimulation may also be caused by emotions and drugs. The dowager with the growling gut at the concert is a case in point. She has had a good, full meal perhaps. Her juices are flowing freely. Her pulse is in repose. She is flushed with social triumph and not pale with fright. The only problem is that her parasympathetic nervous system is pouring out acetylcholine, causing her gut to growl. She may feel short of breath due to contraction of smooth muscle in her bronchial tubes. So, the parasympathetic system is said to be *cholinergic* or *parasympathomimetic*. Cholinergic drugs are relatively few in number. The eye drops used to constrict the pupils in people with glaucoma are cholinergic. The treatment of a certain muscle disorder is with prostigmine, a cholinergic drug.

To go further, one will often see such terms as *antisympathetic,* or *antiparasympathetic,* which mean, simply, against the sympathetic system or parasympathetic system, as the case may be. *Antiadrenergic* or *anticholinergic* are synonyms, respectively, for antisympathetic or antiparasympathetic. If matters are not complicated enough already, one may read of ganglionic blocking agents. Ganglia are collections of nerve cells outside the central nervous system, i.e., outside of the brain and spinal cord. These ganglia are, for the most part, a mixture of sympathetic and parasympathetic cells transmitting their messages by secreting adrenalin-like (adrenergic) or acetylcholine-like (cholinergic) substances. Perhaps the best-known ganglion is the solar plexus which lies, roughly, behind the stomach.

Finally, to keep terms straight, there are anticholinergic agents, i.e., agents that block parasympathetic impulses. *Parasympatholytic* is a synonym for anticholinergic.

Table 4-1 and the following glossary may help to keep matters simple.

Table 4-1   Parasympathetic vs. Sympathetic Effects

Parasympathetic Effects (cholinergic)	Sympathetic Effects (adrenergic)
Pupils constricted for near vision	Pupils dilated for far vision
Heart rate slowed	Heart rate increased
Skin may be flushed	Pallor and "goose bumps"
Salivation may increase	Dry mouth
Bronchial passages may contract	Bronchial passages dilated
May be outpouring of mucus	Flow of mucus diminished
Peristaltic motion increased	Peristaltic motion diminished
Flow of digestive juices increased	Flow of digestive juices diminished
Sweating generally increased	Sweating generally decreased but with nervous sweating of palms, armpits, and crotch.

Central nervous system   That part of the nervous system comprised of the brain and spinal cord.

Autonomic nervous system   The involuntary or self-regulating nervous system.

Adrenergic   Mediated by adrenalin-like substances.

Sympathetic nervous system   That part of the autonomic nervous system that is adrenergic.

Cholinergic   Mediated by acetylcholine-like substances.

Parasympathetic nervous system   That part of the autonomic nervous system that is cholinergic.

Sympathomimetic   Having an adrenergic effect.

Parasympathomimetic   Having a cholinergic effect.

Antiadrenergic (sympatholytic)   Inhibiting or reducing an adrenergic effect.

Anticholinergic (parasympatholytic)   Inhibiting or reducing a cholinergic effect.

Drug actions are not always simple, nor can one action always be separated from another. Different patients may have different responses to drugs. A particular individual may respond to the same drug differently at different times. Old people are much more susceptible to most drug actions than are young people. As a general rule, if a drug has one fairly strong anticholinergic effect it will have another, perhaps unwanted, effect. If a drug has one strong adrenergic effect, it probably will have two or more.

Drugs that influence the autonomic nervous system are mostly adrenergic or anticholinergic. There are relatively few cholinergic drugs and still fewer antiadrenergic drugs, and these have very limited but important use in medicine. Cholinergic eye drops and certain drugs used in cardiovascular diseases are the exception to this rule.

To some extent, we have explained how drugs work by inhibiting or stimulating nerve impulses. Now let's see how drugs work on living cells. It is easy to take a penicillin pill or a sulfa pill for an infection. These agents have saved millions of lives, but they have killed thousands. Many drugs that can kill living organisms, such as bacteria, can kill humans under certain circumstances. This balance between evil and good, kill and cure, is expressed as the *therapeutic index*. In simplified terms, it is the lethal dose (LD) divided by the effective dose (ED), LD/ED. If 1 gram of a drug can help a patient and 2 grams can kill, the therapeutic index is 2. Such a drug may be fairly safe to use were it not for the many symptoms that patients can have and still survive.

For our purpose, let's propose a *safety index* defined by the maximum safe dose (SD) divided by the effective dose (ED). It is then obvious that the safety index is much smaller than the therapeutic index. The safety index is a mathematical expression of the *margin of safety*. If the SD is 2 grams, the ED is 1 gram, and the safety index is 2, the margin of safety is 100 percent. The difficulty is in knowing in advance what figures are since they may vary from person to person, and in the same person as conditions change. For example, the margin of safety of digitalis, a heart medicine, can vary according to the amount of potassium in a patient's blood plasma.

It is well to point out here that most drugs are effective in very small quantities. A gram is one-thousandth of a kilogram, which is 2.2 pounds. A milligram is one-thousandth of a gram or one-millionth of a kilogram. Most drug doses are measured in milligrams. Ten milligrams of morphine will render a normal person stuporous for 4 to 12 hours. Atropine is generally used as a cholinergic blocking agent. In the usual dose of 0.5 milligram, it will dry the mouth, blur the vision, and quiet the gut for half a day.

That one is dealing with very powerful chemicals may explain why they are not well understood. Acetylcholine, adrenalin, and other naturally occurring chemicals are present in such small quantities that their presence cannot be detected except by their action, that is, by bioassay, and that is where we started this chapter. Minced mouse brains are used to assay certain drugs.

Drugs such as insulin and thyroid replace bodily deficiencies. Diabetes is a common disease in old people and can be controlled by insulin, a substance normally secreted by the pancreas, an organ behind the stomach. In diabetes there may be a deficiency of insulin or inability to use the normal amounts of insulin that the pancreas secretes. If a diabetic needs it, insulin derived from swine or cattle can be injected. In old people, the danger of severe reactions is far greater than in young people. Thyroid, also derived from animals, probably has been used promiscuously, as in the case of Mrs. O., but its use can, on occasion, be life-saving.

At this point, a few basic concepts should be stated in greater detail. Drugs either replace something, depress something, or stimulate something. Given as replacement of hormones, such as cortisone, thyroid, or insulin, drugs enter the natural functioning of the body. Other drugs, such as levodopa (used in Parkinson's disease) or vitamins, also replace body deficiencies.

Drugs may actually depress or inhibit something when they seem to stimulate. Diuretics, such as chlorothiazide (Diuril) or furosemide (Lasix), seem to stimulate kidney function. However, the diuretics inhibit enzymes in the kidney tubules that resorb salts into the blood. Because the salts are not resorbed, the water that would be drawn with the salts is not resorbed, and salts and water eventually are excreted in larger amounts.

The action of many drugs is not understood. The manner in which many sedatives, painkillers, and anesthetics work simply is not known. It is known, however, that almost any drug that is inhaled, swallowed, injected, applied, or rubbed in can harm some people, especially old people. A drug may not have a single effect. It may inhibit enzymes in kidney tubules to cause diuresis. It may also have a related action in the ear to cause temporary or permanent deafness. Aspirin acts in one part of the brain to suppress pain, in another part to reduce fever. It reduces the inflammation in arthritic joints. In kidneys, depending on the dose, aspirin may increase or decrease uric acid excretion. It may act on platelets to inhibit blood clotting. In many instances, especially in the brain, drugs have several actions which may or may not cause a desirable balance of effects. An illustration of a drug having a combination of effects is the propensity of certain antibiotics to both inhibit bacteria and cause deafness. Other drugs may relieve inward nervousness and cause frightful tremors at the same time. The tendence of evil to mingle with good is like a pharmacological morality play, bizarre and unfathomable.

In the young person the actions of a drug may be limited; the primary action initiates a secondary response to maintain a certain balance. In the old, this balance is impaired, and small alterations may throw a delicate chemical balance out of equilibrium. As people get older, their tissues, enzymes, and body composition change. The body is less able to regulate itself and to adjust to drug actions. Drugs do exactly the same things at the cellular level in the old person as in the young, but because of changes in the quantity and quality of substances on which the drugs act, the sum or balance of effects is changed to produce results which may be exaggerated, diminished, or even paradoxical.

EFFECTS OF DRUGS ON THE ELDERLY

Now let us consider in greater detail why the elderly have a disproportionate share of problems with drugs. One hospital-based survey of general medical patients found that persons over 80 years old had a nearly 25 percent incidence of side effects from drugs, while those under 50 years had less than a 12 percent incidence of side effects.[1] Another study found a sevenfold difference in side effects between those in their twenties and seventies.[2] Problems often result from the following factors associated with aging: (1) more chronic illnesses requiring more potent drugs, (2) changing homeostatic balances in the aging body, and (3) changing pharmacokinetics. We shall now review these matters:

1 Although those over 65 years constitute only about 10 percent of the population of the United States, they consume about 25 to 28 percent of the drugs, meaning they take 3 to 3½ times as many drugs as their juniors. The more drugs, the more problems they cause—not in direct proportion to their increased use, but at an exponential rate. Drugs often interact with each other, causing increased or decreased intensity or duration of effect. Although there are relatively few symptomatic interactions in younger people, unpleasant reactions are frequent in older persons.

The greater drug use in the elderly is a reflection of two facts: (1) increased incidence of illness and (2) the disturbing tendency of physicians to overmedicate their patients. These facts are especially true in chronic illnesses such as arthritis, cardiovascular diseases, and psychiatric problems.

2 The second factor, which is somewhat related to the first, is altered homeostatic mechanisms in the older person. As one ages, a fragile balance among many factors may be lost, and drugs may have untoward effects.

3 The next major change with aging relates not to what the drug does to the person but what the person does to the drug. These are the pharmacokinetic changes, i.e., how fast and to what extent the body absorbs, distributes, metabolizes, and eventually excretes the drug. These factors determine the degree and duration of the drug action.

A DRUG IN THE BODY: SEQUENCE OF EVENTS

We shall now consider what happens when a person uses an oral medication. After a person swallows a tablet or capsule, it disintegrates in the stomach. If the drug is alkaline, stomach acid converts it to a salt as the drug dissolves, and it ionizes. Because drugs are not generally absorbed in the ionized state, alkaline drugs are primarily absorbed into the body in the more alkaline environment of the small intestine, where they revert to an un-ionized state. Acidic drugs, such as aspirin, which are un-ionized in the stomach, are absorbed there more readily. Because of the greater absorbing surface in the folds and mircroscopic projections of the small intestine, however, much absorption of acidic drugs occurs there also.

Absorption, the passage of drugs from the intestine to the blood stream, occurs by one or more mechanisms for any given drug: (1) *passive diffusion* across the membranes; (2) *convective absorption*, in which the substance is moved along with the movement of fluids; (3) *active transport* involving *ion-pair transport*, in which sulfonic acids and complex ammonium compounds combine with substances in the gastrointestinal tract and then passively diffuse into the blood; and (4) *pinocytosis*, the engulfment of oils or solid particles and their transfer across the intestinal wall to lymphatic and venous capillaries.

It should now be apparent that a number of factors affect the rate of absorption. Among these are (1) the degree of stomach acidity, (2) how rapidly the stomach empties its contents into the small intestine, (3) how rapidly materials pass through the small intestine, (4) how much mixing in the intestine occurs to bring drugs into contact with absorbing surfaces, (5) the quantities of carriers, and (6) the vascularity and blood flow at the absorption sites.

Hydrochloric acid secretion in the stomach declines with age. This decline alters the solubility and ionization of drugs and hence the degree and rate of their absorption. In old people, absorption may be impaired by reduced peristaltic activity in the gastrointestinal (GI) tract. Reduced blood flow to the GI tract may also impair absorption.[1] Old people have fewer absorbing cells in the intestine, leading to impaired absorption. Decreased phosphorylation (a chemical reaction) in the intestinal lining delays absorption of galactose, a simple sugar. Absorption of xylose, another sugar, decreases 40 percent as one ages from 18 to 80 years.[3]

The drug is then *distributed*. It first enters the portal circulation and passes through the liver, where it may be changed by enzymes. This is known as the "first-pass effect" and may cause a number of drugs to lose much of their potency. (Naturally, this effect is not present when drugs are injected.) From the liver, the drug enters the systemic circulation. Then it may be bound to proteins in the blood or to tissues. It may enter cells, be dispersed in body water, or accumulate in high concentrations in certain organs or tissues. A fat-soluble drug may dissolve to some degree in body fat. The extent to which any of these processes occurs may vary greatly from drug to drug or from person to person.

The extent to which blood proteins, mainly albumin and globulin, bind a drug largely determines how much and how long it will act. Only the unbound (free) drug is active and metabolized. If a drug is highly bound, say 90 percent, it takes only a small increase in the unbound portion to exert a much greater action. For example, by increasing the free portion from 4 to 6 percent, there is a 50 percent increase in the effective blood level. On the other hand, for a poorly bound drug, an increase of 2 percent in the unbound portion is not much at all.

Reduced quantities of blood proteins can cause higher levels and faster excretion of certain drugs. The few studies on the effects of age, per se, on protein binding are contradictory.[4,5]

The total systemic blood flow decreases with age.[6] The ratios of total body fluid to lean cell mass and of blood volume to body weight remain constant, but after the age of 19 cardiac output declines about 1 percent each year.[7-9] A reduced proportion of of the remaining flow goes to the liver and the kidneys, the metabolizing and excreting organs, and more goes to the brain and the heart muscle.[6]

Assuming a constant body weight, body fat increases with age. The male teenager is 18 percent fat, and by the time he is 85 he is about 36 percent fat. During this same period, women increase from 33 to 45 percent fat. Still assuming weight remains constant, there is a proportionate decline in lean cell mass and blood volume. As a result, all other things being equal, a given dose of a drug should produce a higher blood level because it is dispersed in a smaller volume. But all other things are not equal: (1) drugs generally are absorbed more slowly in old people and (2) after absorption, some drugs are stored in the increased body fat. Both these factors may limit the rise in the blood level of a drug and, thus, its action.[10]

We now consider another pharmacokinetic concept, the *volume of distribution* (Vd) of a drug. The volume of distribution is not the volume of a person's body nor of his or her blood volume, but the hypothetical volume in which a given dose of a drug would be dispersed if its concentration in the entire body were the same as its concentration in the blood. This volume, which will vary with each drug, is found by dividing the dose of a drug by the blood concentration of the drug. For instance, let us assume that we inject 1000 milligrams of a drug into a person's vein, wait a few minutes to allow the drug to become evenly dispersed in the blood, and then withdraw a sample of blood and analyze it. Let's suppose that the analysis gives 1 milligram per 100 milliliters. Then the volume of distribution is

$$Vd = \frac{1000 \text{ mg}}{1 \text{ mg}/100 \text{ ml}} = 100,000 \text{ ml or } 100 \text{ liters}$$

This high volume of distribution (a person's blood volume is typically 5 to 6 liters) indicates that much of the drug is in other body organs and fat, and that relatively little is in the blood. If we repeat the process with another drug and find a concentration of 15 milligrams per 100 milliliters of blood, the Vd is 6.7 liters, and we can assume the drug is mostly in the blood and little is in other body tissues.

The distribution of a drug throughout the body depends on a number of factors. Among these are the drug's solubility in body fluids and in fat; its binding by blood proteins and by body tissues and organs, such as the liver and the brain; and its ability to penetrate tissue barriers such as those protecting the brain, spinal cord, and placenta. Several tissues and organs have claims on each drug, and the Vd represents the blood's claim to that drug. It is not surprising, therefore, that an increase in proportion of body fat, a decline in blood volume by the same ratio, and a reduction in cell mass in other tissues, such as the brain, result in a change in the Vd and, therefore, a change in the blood level of a drug from a given dose. A drug with a relatively low volume of distribution in a healthy young person (meaning most of the drug is in the blood) will have an even lower Vd in an old person.

From the time drugs are absorbed, they may be undergoing *metabolism* to either an active or inactive form. Metabolism here is, in general, a process which converts substances in the blood into a form which can be excreted more readily. Some drugs are excreted unchanged while others are combined or conjugated with substances or are broken apart chemically. Moreover, not all drugs are active in the form in which they are administered but must be metabolically converted to be active. Drug metabolism occurs principally in the liver, but may also occur in the intestinal wall during absorption, in the kidneys, in muscles, and in blood.

A number of drugs, including antipyrine, phenylbutazone, aminopyrine, indomethacin, and amobarbital are metabolized more slowly in the elderly, but this slowing may be caused by reduced blood flow to the metabolizing enzymes of the liver rather than by a decline in the metabolizing enzymes themselves.

Drugs which are not rapidly excreted are generally quite lipid-soluble. Their duration of action, therefore, is limited by their change to an excretable form. Although there may be some decline in the activity of metabolizing enzymes as one ages, the reserve capacity of the liver is so great that there is probably little change in their action as one gets older. This decline is also a relative pheonomenon. For instance, acetaminophen is usually metabolized much faster in younger persons, but old fast metabolizers still metabolize it faster than young slow metabolizers.[11]

Finally, the drug is *excreted*. There is some small amount of excretion through the saliva, lungs, sweat, and milk. The main excretory routes are through the kidneys and gastrointestinal tract. Drugs excreted through the gastrointestinal tract are removed from the blood in the liver, pass through the bile duct to the intestine, and are excreted. Some substances may be resorbed and recycled from gut to blood to liver to gut. There may also be some diffusion from blood across the intestinal wall to the lumen of the intestine.

In urinary excretion, substances in the blood may be filtered through the glomeruli of the kidneys and pass through the tubules, kidney pelvis, and ureter to the bladder. How rapidly this mechanism works depends on the volume of blood flow to the kidneys and the number of their functioning units called nephrons, each of which consists of glomerulus and its tubules. Narrowing of the renal vasculature and decreased cardiac output cause a 50 percent decline in renal plasma flow as one ages from 20 to 90 years.[12] Tubular mass and glomerular filtration rate, the volume of blood filtering through the glomeruli per unit of time—each decline about 45 percent from age 20 to 90, or about 6 percent every 10 years. The young adult's kidneys filter about 200 liters of blood every 24 hours to produce about 1500 milliliters of urine. An old person's filters about 120 liters to produce about 1000 milliliters of urine. Individual nephrons simply stop functioning rather than decline gradually.[13-16]

SUMMARY

The material reviewed here is simplified but may be studied in more detail in any standard textbook or review of physiology and pharmacology. Our aim is, as has been stated, to give the general reader an idea of what drugs do in the body. In following chapters we shall return to these fundamentals as we discuss particular drugs in greater detail.

Drug reactions are much more common than most people appreciate. This is the topic of the next chapter.

REFERENCES

1   L. G. Seidl et al., "Studies on the Epidemiology of Adverse Drug Reactions: III Reactions in Patients on a General Medical Service," *Bull. John Hopkins Hosp.* **119**:299–315(1966).

2   N. Hurwitz, "Predisposing Factors in Adverse Drug Reactions," *Br. Med. J.* **1**:536–539(1969).

3   M. Essam Fikry and M. H. Aboul-Wafa, "Intestinal Absorption in the Old," *Gerontol. Clin.* **7**:171–178(1965).

4   Edward J. Triggs & Roger L. Nation, "Pharmacokinetics in the Aged: A Review," *J. Pharmacokinet. and Biopharm* **3**:387–418(1973).

5   Douglas A. Bender et al., "Plasma Protein Binding of Drugs as a Function of Age in Adult Human Subjects," *J. Pharm. Sci* **64**:1711–1713(1975).

6   Douglas A. Bender, "A Pharmacodynamic Basis for Changes in Drug Activity Associated with Aging in the Adult," *Exp. Gerontol.* **1**:237–247(1967).

7   Nathan W. Shock, "Physiological Aspects of Aging in Man," *Annu. Rev. Physiol.* **23**:97–122(1961).

8   W. A. Ritschel, "Pharmacokinetic Approach to Drug Dosing in the Aged," *J. Am. Geriatr. Soc.* **24**:344–354(1976).

9   Douglas A. Bender, "The Effect of Increasing Age on the Distribution of Peripheral Blood Flow in Man," *J. Am. Geriatr. Soc.* **13**:192–198(1965).

10 Ladislav P. Novak, "Total Body Potassium, Fat Free Mass, Cell Mass in Males and Females between the Ages 18 and 85 years," *J. Gerontol.* **27**:438–443(1972).

11 Robin Brian et al., "Rate of Acetaminophen Metabolism in the Elderly and the Young," *J. Am. Geriatr. Soc.* **28**:339(1976).

12 John Bland, "Regulation of Fluid and Electrolyte Balance in Aged Persons," *J. Am. Geriatr. Soc.* **1**:233–243(1963).

13 Charles H. Heider and Albert N. Brest, "Renal Insufficiency in the Aged," *Geriatrics* **18**:489–493(1963).

14 A. D. Mitchell and William L. Velk, "Renal Function in the Aged," *Geriatrics* **8**:263–266(1953).

15 Sidney Vernon, "Nocturia in the Elderly Male," *J. Am. Geriatr. Soc.* **6**:411–414(1958).

16 Dean F. Davies and Nathan W. Shock, "Age Changes in the Glomerular Filtration Rate, Effective Renal Plasma Flow, and Tubular Excretory Capacity in Adult Males," *J. Clin. Invest.* **29**:496–507(1950).

Chapter 5

Undesirable Drug Effects

It is not our aim here to make a catalog of drug-related symptoms. Rather we wish to tell you how such symptoms have come to our attention so often. Our experience has led to a wariness in prescribing, which we believe is thoroughly justified. We hope that this chapter will lead some of our colleagues to question, to hesitate, to be alert, and to be suspicious when it comes to diagnosing and treating old people.

Error in the prescribing of drugs occurs much more often than is generally appreciated. Assuming that drugs are properly manufactured and stored (not always a safe assumption, by the way), the prescribing physician has the first opportunity for error. Not long ago, for example, a nurse questioned one of us about a dose of an anticonvulsant a physician had ordered by telephone for an elderly lady. Had the nurse not been alert, a patient could have been killed. The point is that physicians, all physicians, may make mistakes. Drugs are so numerous that no physician can remember the proper dose for all of them. This is why physicians should use mainly the relatively few drugs they understand well and not attempt to use or try every drug available.

Physicians may err while under constant pressure to do something. To some physicians, nurses, and relatives the well-treated patient is the quiet, uncomplaining patient. For example, it is intolerable to some night-duty nurses for a patient to be awake. The nurse may awaken the physician to put someone else to sleep when kind words and reassurance would serve as well as a sedative. It is unfortunate that some nurses believe that their chief function is to give medicines. Some abuse their discretionary authority when medicines are ordered *prn* (*pro re nata*, or as necessary.) The nurse may do better for patients by questioning their need for medication than by giving it mindlessly on a set schedule.

The practice of pharmacy has greatly improved in the last 20 years or so. Pharmacists have become better informed, better trained, and more professional in their approach. Their job should include questioning, monitoring, and educating. We have found that by working together—nurse, physician, and pharmacist—mistakes can be kept to a minimum. We shall have more to say about this relationship in a later chapter.

In addition to doctors, pharmacists, and nurses, one must consider that patients and their families may make many mistakes in drug use. One clinical study showed that about 60 percent of elderly, self-sufficient outpatients made medication errors. Among these mistakes were discontinuing medicines, taking improper doses, or taking them at the wrong times or in the wrong sequence.

Patients' mistakes may be due to a number of causes. Among these may be a poor understanding of the purpose of a medicine. The pharmacist and the physician should be explicit. They should explain. They should reiterate. They should make sure they are understood. If patients are deaf, confused, cannot read directions, or take a number of different medicines, mistakes are much more apt to occur. If patients are poor or depressed they may, unknown to the physician, not get their prescriptions filled.

It should go without saying—but needs to be said—that the fewer the number of medicines, the fewer reactions and errors. Having considered what people do with drugs, let's now consider what drugs may do to people.

How frequent are undesirable or dangerous drug reactions? The general belief is that they are rare or infrequent. With warnings of the Food and Drug Administration to protect people and the frequent admonition for patients to "ask your doctor," we are lulled into a sense of false security. In our geriatrics practice, we have found that for each prescription there is always a chance of an unfavorable reaction of some sort. One study of hospitalized patients found that among patients over 80 there was about a 25 percent incidence of adverse drug reactions. Another study showed that old people had about seven times as many bad reactions as people under 40.

Some dangerous drug reactions may not be suspected because the symptoms may be attributed to old age. For example, a mild sedative has, on occasion, caused a feeble old person to be even more unsteady on her (most often) already unsteady feet. A resultant fall might cause a hip fracture for which the medicine might never be blamed or even suspected.

If one remembers that the average person over 65 takes an average of four drugs, the potential for harm is enormous. Laxatives, headache remedies, sedatives, tranquilizers, antidepressants, salves, antiseptics, enemas, antacids, antibiotics, and other drugs are presumed by some to be innocuous. They are frequently used without prescription, and are considered by many people not to be drugs at all.

The problem is compounded when one considers that drug reactions can be, and most often are, identical to symptoms of disease. When confronted with an ill old person who has taken a number of medicines, it is often necessary to discontinue the medicines to assess symptoms. In a surprising number of cases, the patient will improve, as did Mrs. O. It is unfortunate that too many physicians have a tendency to prescribe medicine to relieve symptoms caused by medicine. Sometimes treating medicine with medicine works; at times there is no other reasonable course of action, but such treatment is expensive and complicated.

We can state categorically that drug reactions are among the most frequent causes of symptoms in old people. What are some of the symptoms? What does one look for? Let's make rounds at the Methodist Homes where the authors formerly worked together. Old people living here are *residents*, who live in rooms and apartments with a moderate amount of independence and *patients*, who depend on continuing nursing and medical care. Residents can take their own medicines and go and come when they please; patients require that a nurse or nurse-assistant administer drugs.

One of us was called because Mrs. J. had fainted in her own quarters, a frequent but always frightful event in the life of an old person. Fortunately she had not fallen and broken a bone. After lengthy examination and questioning, it came out that she had taken a dose of Epsom salt. The resulting shift in her body water, inside and outside her bowel, had caused her to faint. Her swoon possibly could have been fatal.

What other medicines might have caused faintness? Sedatives, tranquilizers, certain heart medicines, antibiotics that may have a laxative effect, laxatives, aspirin, or other pain-relieving drugs. Of course, any number of abnormal states can also cause giddiness, faintness, falls, seizures, or turns.

Mrs. B. developed bruised patches on her limbs. Of course, old skin is thinner and less resilient than young skin, but the symptom was new to Mrs. B. After considering a number of causes, it developed that Mrs. B. had been taking Butazolidin, frequently used for arthritis. Butazolidin inhibits platelets and, therefore, increases the tendency toward easy bruising, which already exists in old people.

Certain antibiotics, painkillers, sedatives, laxatives, sulfa drugs, i.e., almost any drug can cause a skin rash in a sensitive person. Among these are Ex-Lax, Feen-a-mint, and Alophen, frequently used laxatives which can be bought without perscription.

For years, Mr. S. had taken a blood-thinning medicine for heart trouble. (To be technical, blood thinners don't thin the blood, but they do enhance the bleeding tendency.) He went to an orthopedist for treatment of a painful knee. The doctor prescribed Butazolidin, not knowing or inquiring about other medicines Mr. S. was taking. The interaction between the blood thinner and the arthritis medicine brought on a serious hemorrhage from the bowel requiring hospitalization and transfusion treatment.

Blood thinners are dangerous and we believe their use in elderly patients should be seriously questioned. We have seen serious brain hemorrhage on at least two occasions apparently caused by blood thinners. In addition, we have seen hemorrhage from the gastrointestinal system or the urinary system a dozen times or more. We shall discuss drug interactions at greater length later.

Mrs. W. had been depressed and was given an antidepressant. It caused her to have a dry nose and mouth, and she chose to fight her depression without medicine. Atropine and a long list of similar drugs (anticholinergic drugs) can cause dryness of the mucous membranes, constipation, urinary retention, dryness of the skin, and blurring of the vision. Several tranquilizers and antidepressant drugs have this anticholinergic action which we explained in the last chapter.

Stomach cramps are frequently treated with a mixture of a sedative and an anticholinergic drug. Such drugs, then, can cause some or all the symptoms mentioned in the preceding paragraph.

Mr. V. had a cold. He was given a decongestant, which helped his cold by reducing the amount of water and mucus in his nose. It also constipated him, made it impossible for him to pass his urine, and blurred his vision because of its anticholinergic action. He recovered from his cold much faster than he recovered from 2 days' (four capsules) treatment for it.

The manner in which drugs are promoted and sold can contribute to the problem of drug misuse. Bold letters proclaim the benefits of a drug or preparation. Photographs, often with sexual overtones, suggest that we too can attain the ideal state pictured therein if we use a particular product. But what of the warnings? The side effects? Look to the fine print: drowsiness, confusion, nausea, skin rash, slurred speech, etc., etc. In old people especially the dangers from using a drug may just be greater than any possible benefit.

Recently, Mr. L., an elderly, confused, disoriented man, came to our care. He could not walk. His speech was slurred. There was a history of alcoholism. Any of his symptoms could be ascribed to a chronic organic brain syndrome, fairly common in very old people. It did come out that this old patient had been taking Valium for weeks while hospitalized. As he gradually discontinued its use, his condition improved, he could dress himself, and he could relate to others, though still disabled because of his brain disease.

Physicians—good, wise, and intelligent as they may be—are subject to psychological pressures and often do not appreciate the fine print. It is easier to prescribe a tranquilizer than to listen as a person relates a woeful tale. Physicians are pressed in our drugged society to prescribe and, rightly, assume that if they don't, someone else will. Maybe the handful of geriatricians appreciate more than others the harm such attitudes can cause.

Constipation, blurred vision, urinary incontinence, and others are just some of the symptoms shared by many drugs and are not at all uncommon. And as is coming increasingly to light, some drugs, like Valium for example, in susceptible persons are habit-forming. They can cause serious effects if misused, as suggested by the "side effects" indicated in the fine print.

The fineness of print on some advertisements would lead one to believe that the adverse reactions are negligible, when as a matter of fact one could almost say that, with many drugs, if there are no side effects the drug may not be giving full benefit. In other words, side effects and benefits are often inseparable.

Many of the antidepressant drugs have subtle effects. One of the most frequently used is amitriptyline. An elderly patient of ours has taken it for about 20 years, since it first became available. He is habituated to it—though addiction is not listed as one of its dangers—or at least he will not or cannot stop taking it. Among its adverse reactions are excitement, anxiety, restlessness, numbness, tingling, and paresthesia of the extremities, incoordination, dry mouth, constipation, etc., etc. Our patient has all these symptoms but he refuses to believe that any of them could be due to medicine he has taken for over 20 years. "It never caused me any trouble before," he says, as if that exonerates the medicine now that he is 77. One wonders if he could not have had a much more comfortable old age if he had endured his depression without medicine long ago.

A frequent occurrence is for a constipating medicine to be taken concurrently with a laxative. As a routine, belladonna, the most frequently prescribed anticholinergic agent, may be prescribed for gastrointestinal cramps or bladder spasms. It is a very constipating drug. Patients frequently end up taking a laxative for drug-induced sluggishness of the bowel.

This discussion of drug-induced symptoms has been presented in a random fashion. To summarize, there is scarcely a symptom anyone can have that cannot be induced unpredictably in a susceptible person by some drug. Let's start at the top and go down. Baldness of a particular kind may be due to a drug called Benemid. Ringing in the ears may be caused by aspirin. Blurred vision may be caused by hundreds of drugs that influence the eyes. Glaucoma, a common disease in the elderly which can cause blindness, is aggravated by many drugs, including the antihistamines in over-the-counter cold and cough medicines.

Certain aminoglycoside antibiotics can cause deafness. Dryness of nose and mouth and palpitation are caused by many drugs, especially adrenergic drugs. Asthma can be caused or greatly aggravated by Inderal, a very useful drug for certain heart and blood-pressure disorders.

Gas, constipation, and diarrhea may be caused by any number of medicines. Some drugs even can produce an effect resembling an acute abdominal surgical emergency. Certain antibiotics have caused severe ulceration of the bowel resembling a very serious disease called chronic ulcerative colitis.

The kidney is susceptible to severe reactions. The phenacetin in many highly advertised painkillers has caused many cases of kidney damage in long-term users. A number of antibiotics that are used almost promiscuously can kill people or destroy their kidneys. A large number of other drugs endanger kidney function.

The liver is susceptible to damage by literally hundreds of drugs. Among them is chlorpromazine, one of the most frequently used drugs for psychiatric disorders.

The marrow and lymphoid organs that make the components of blood are influenced by all classes of drugs. Chloramphenicol, an otherwise excellent antibiotic, has its usefulness limited because it caused several hundred, if not several thousand, deaths before its dangers were fully appreciated.

Drugs can and do cause some truly horrendous and lasting harm to the nervous system. Alcohol does more harm nationwide than any other drug and its abuse has been dealt with by physicians, writers, and reformers for many years. A number of antipsychotic drugs cause tardive dyskinesia, a grotesque jerkiness of tongue, lips, and jaw. Compazine, an antiemetic, on occasion can cause frightful jerkiness of the neck muscles that make its use questionable.

The skin can develop all kinds of bizarre eruptions as a result of drugs. *Epidermolysis bullosa*, a severe and often fatal skin eruption, has resulted from drugs that were considered to be innocuous.

The problem is not simple. The overuse, misuse, and abuse of drugs is a national health problem. The control machinery has, for the most part, been installed. For certain drugs an awareness of the scope of the problem is necessary to contain it, and that is what we are trying to stimulate.

The problem is, of course, aggravated exponentially when a person takes several drugs, as most old people do. Drugs not only act on people, they act on each other. Drug interations can be very complex, and this is what we'll now discuss.

Most informed people are aware of the potentiating effects ethyl alcohol and most sedatives have on each other. It is sobering to consider the prevalence of the use of each. By no means is this the only instance of one class of drug augmenting the action of another. We have mentioned the augmentation of blood thinners by phenylbutazone (Butazolidin), and there are hundreds more.

Only a few years ago a group of drugs called monoamine oxidase (MAO, an enzyme that destroys naturally occurring adrenergic substances) inhibitors were found to be useful in treating depression. It soon became apparent that such drugs made it extremely dangerous to eat cheese, sour cream, chocolate, chicken livers, or even pickled herring. These foods have a high content of tyramine, a precursor of certain monoamines which have marked adrenergic effects. This is an extreme example of how enzyme inhibition can work.

When one considers the sheer number of prescriptions some people take, it is no wonder that harmful drug interations are increasing. The medical profession has not, in our experience, been as sensitive as it should be in trying to prevent such interactions. Perhaps this lack of sensitivity is due to what Butler calls the "old age write-off." Simply put, this condescending procedure occurs when a physician writes a prescription instead of making a conscientious effort to make an accurate diagnosis and treat appropriately.

Table 5-1 points out some of the pharmacological mechanisms that lead to undesirable drug interactions. For example, a person may be taking an antacid for a hiatus hernia, a common disorder in old people. The person might then

Table 5-1   Mechanisms and Examples of Drug Interactions

Pharmacological mechanisms	Examples of pharmacological mechanisms
Absorption	Aluminum hydroxide interferes with absorption of tetracycline.
Possible cross-allergenicity	Cephalosporins with penicillin.
Increased or diminished excretion	Thiazide diuretics predispose patient to digitalis toxicity through loss of potassium in urine.
Metabolic conflicts	Coumarins increase metabolism of barbiturates.
Plasma protein binding	Sulfonamides diminish plasma protein binding of phenylbutazone.
Mucosal irritation	Aspirin added to phenylbutazone irritates stomach more than either drug alone.
Competition for receptor sites	Methyldopa diminishes number of receptor sites for adrenergic drugs and for other antihypertensive drugs.
Pharmacologic effect increased or decreased	Alcohol increases effect of barbiturates. Tricyclic antidepressants decrease effect of propranolol.

develop a urinary infection for which tetracycline is prescribed. It is not sufficiently appreciated that tetracycline requires a slightly acid medium in the stomach for absorption. The antacid then counteracts to some extent the possible benefit of tetracycline. This, then, is an example of the effect one drug may have on the absorption of another.

To the credit of the pharmaceutical manufacturers, some of them are genuinely interested in the welfare of patients. We are indebted to Lederle Laboratories for Table 5-2, which outlines the more serious drug interactions. Such interactions sometimes have required chemical detective work for their understanding.

SUMMARY

It has not been our purpose here to consider all adverse drug interactions, but we have told of some of the most flagrant. For those who want to consider this fascinating topic more extensively, we suggest the book by P. D. Hansten, *Drug Interactions*.

We have mentioned that laxatives and anticholinergics can have antagonistic effects, i.e., one medicine cancels the effect of the other to some extent.

A thiazide diuretic is often used in patients with congestive heart failure who take digitalis. The diuretic may cause excessive excretion of potassium. Potassium depletion then may cause digitalis toxicity. When the patient becomes much sicker, it is often difficult to sort out the cause for his or her plight. It then becomes mandatory to discontinue both medicines cautiously to assess the situation.

We have pointed out that drug reactions may be blatant, obscure, confusing, insidious, and subtle. They may occur because of carelessness or ignorance. They are more frequent than most people realize, even the victims.

We have suggested that the prevention of harmful reactions in old people should engage the attention of physicians, nurses, pharmacists, and patients and their families.

In the next few chapters we shall discuss classes of drugs according to their main uses or according to organ systems. We shall begin with gastrointestinal drugs.

Table 5-2 Particularly Critical Drug Interactions

Primary drug	Interacting agent	Potentially dangerous effect
	Oral anticoagulants	
(Dicumarol, Coumadin, Panwarfin, Athrombin-K)	Anabolic and androgenic steroids (Anadrol, Androyd, Dianabol)	Increased anticoagulant effects
	Barbiturates (Nembutal, Seconal, Butisol)	Decreased anticoagulant effects
	Chloral hydrate (Noctec, Felsules)	Increase anticoagulant effects
	Chloramphenicol (Chloromycetin, Amphicol)	Increased anticoagulant effects
	Clofibrate (Atromid-S)	Increased anticoagulant effects
	Dextrothyroxine (Choloxin)	Increased anticoagulant effects
	Disulfiram (Antabuse)	Increased anticoagulant effects
	Glutethimide (Doriden)	Decreased anticoagulant effects
	Oxyphenbutazone (Tandearil) Phenylbutazone (Butazolidin) Indomethacin (Indocin)	Increased anticoagulant effects
	Salicylates	Increased antigoagulant effects
	Sulfonylureas (Orinase, Diabinese, Tolinase, Dymelor)	Increased anticoagulant and hypoglycemic effects
	Thyroid hormones	Increased anticoagulant effects
	Phenytoin (Dilantin)	Increased phenytoin toxicity
	Tricyclic antidepressants	
(Tofranil, Elavil, Etrafon, Pertofrane, Aventyl, Vivactil, Sinequan)	Guanethidine (Ismelin)	Decreased hypotensive effects; hypertensive crisis
	MAO inhibitors (Nardil, Parnate, Eutonyl, Marplan, Furoxone)	Hyperpyrexia convulsions

(continued)

Primary drug	Interacting agent	Potentially dangerous effect
	Sympathomimetic amines (amphetamines, ephedrine, Isuprel, Ritalin, Sudafed)	Hypertensive crisis
Antimicrobials		
Chloramphenicol (chloromycetin, Amphicol)	Phenytoin (Dilantin)	Increased phenytoin toxicity
	Sulfonylureas (Orinase, Diabinese, Tolinase, Dymelor)	Increased hypoglycemic effects
	Oral anticoagulants (Dicumarol, Coumadin, Panwarfin, Athrombin-K)	Increased anticoagulant effects
Nalidixic acid (NegGram)	Oral anticoagulants	Increased anticoagulant effects
Long-acting sulfonamides	Oral anticoagulants	Increased anticoagulant effects
	Sulfonylureas	Increased hypoglycemic effects
Cardiovascular agents		
Digitalis	Thiazide diuretics (Diuril, Enduron, Hygroton, Renese)	Digitalis toxicity, cardiac arrhythmias
	Sympathomimetic amines (amphetamines, ephedrine, Isuprel, Ritalin, Sudafed)	Increased tendency to cardiac arrhythmias
	Reserpine	Cardiac arrhythmias
Guanethidine (Ismelin)	Tricyclic antidepressants (Tofranil, Elavil, Etrafon, Pertofrane)	Loss of hypotensive effects, hypertensive crisis
	MAO inhibitors (Nardil, Parnate, Eutonyl, Marplan)	Decreased hypotensive effects, hypertensive crisis
	Hypoglycemics (insulin, DBI, Orinase, Diabinese, Dymelor)	Increased hypoglycemia

Reserpine	
Tricyclic antidepressants, MAO inhibitors, sympathomimetic amines	Potentially severe hypertensive effects
Propranolol (Inderal)	Potential congestive heart failure
Digitalis	Cardiac arrhythmias

Thiazide diuretics
(Diuril, HydroDiuril, Hygroton, Enduron, Renese, Naturetin)

Corticosteroids (Aristocort, Celestone, Cortef, Decadron, Medrol, Kenacort)	Enhanced potassium loss, hypokalemia
Digitalis	Increased digitalis toxicity, cardiac arrhythmias
Hypoglycemics (insulin, DBI, Orinase, Diabinese, Dymelor)	Hyperglycemia and glycosuria

Sulfonylurea hypoglycemics
(Orinase, Diabinese, Dymelor, Tolinase)

Oral anticoagulants (Dicumarol, Coumadin)	Increased anticoagulant and hypoglycemic effect
Anabolic steroids (Anadrol, Androyd, Dianabol)	Increased hypoglycemic effects
Chloramphenicol (Chloromycetin)	Increased hypoglycemic effects
Guanethidine (Ismelin)	Increased hypoglycemic effects
MAO inhibitors (Nardil, Parnate, Eutonyl, Marplan)	Increased hypoglycemic effects
Phenylbutazone and oxphenbutazone (Butazolidin, Tandearil)	Increased hypoglycemic effects
Propranolol (Inderal)	Increased hypoglycemic effects
Salicylates	Increased hypoglycemic effects
Long-acting sulfonamides (Sulla)	Increased hypoglycemic effects
Thiazide diuretics (Diuril, Naturetin, Hygroton)	Hypoglycemia and glycosuria

(continued)

35

Primary drug	Interacting agent	Potentially dangerous effect
MAO inhibitors		
(Nardil, Parnate, Eutonyl, Marplan	Levodopa (Dopa, Larodopa)	Hypertensive crisis
	Meperidine (Demerol)	Hypertension, or hypotension and coma/convulsions, impaired ventilation
		Hyperpyrexia, convulsions
	Tricyclic antidepressants (Tofranil, Elavil, Sinequan, Etrafon, Pertofrane, Aventyl, Vivactil)	Hypertensive crisis
	Tyramine (in certain foods and alcoholic beverages—aged cheeses, Chianti wines, beer, sherry, pickled herring, chocolate)	Hypertensive crisis
	Sympathomimetic amines (amphetamines, ephedrine, Isuprel, Ritalin, Levophed, Sudafed, and many appetite-suppressant agents)	
	sulfonylureas (Orinase, Diabinese, Tolinase, Dymelor)	Increased hypoglycemic effects
	Guanethidine (Ismelin)	Decreased hypotensive effects, hypertensive crisis
	Reserpine	Potentially severe hypertensive effects
Sympathomimetic amines		
(Amphetamines, ephedrine, epinephrine, Isuprel, Ritalin, Levophed, Sudafed, and many appetite-suppressing agents canorexics)	Tricyclic antidepressants (Tofranil, Elavil, Etrafon, Sinequan, Pertofrane)	Hypertensive crisis
	Digitalis	Enhanced tendency to cardiac arrhythmias
	MAO inhibitors (Nardil, Parnate Eutonyl, Marplan, Furoxone)	Hypertensive crisis

Sedatives and Tranquilizers

Barbiturates (Nembutal, Seconal, Luminal, Butisol)	Oral anticoagulants (Dicumarol, Coumadin)	Decreased anticoagulant effects
	Alcohol	Enhanced CNS depression
	Minor and major tranquilizers	Enhanced CNS depression
Chloral hydrate (Noctec)	Oral anticoagulants	Increased anticoagulant effects
	Alcohol	Enhanced sedation, prolonged hypnotic effect
Glutethimide (Doriden)	Oral anticoagulants	Decreased anticoagulant effects
Minor tranquilizers (Librium, Valium, Serax, meprobamate)	Alcohol	Enhanced sedation
	Barbiturates	Additive sedative effects
	MAO inhibitors	Enhanced sedation
	Phenothiazines (Thorazine, Mellaril, Compazine)	Additive sedative effects
	Tricyclic antidepressants	Additive sedative effects
Major tranquilizers (Thorazine, Mellaril, Compazine and other phenothiazines)	Antihistamines (Benadryl, Chlor-Trimeton, Coricidin, Dramamine, Phenergan)	Additive sedative effects
	Antihypertensives (other than guanethidine)	Potentiation of hypotensive effects, severe hypotension
	Barbiturates	Enhanced sedation
	Minor tranquilizers	Additive sedative effects
	Narcotic analgesics (Demerol, Percodan, codeine, morphine)	Enhanced sedative effects
	Tricyclic antidepressants	Additive sedative effects

Miscellaneous drugs

| Levodopa (Dopa, Larodopa) | MAO inhibitors (Nardil, Parnate, Eutonyl, Marplan) | Hypertensive crisis |

(continued)

Primary drug	Interacting agent	Potentially dangerous effect
Phenytoin (Dilantin)	Alcohol	Enhanced anticonvulsant effect with acute intoxication
	Chloramphenicol (Chloromycetin)	Increased phenytoin toxicity
	Oral anticoagulants	Increased phenytoin toxicity
	Isoniazid (Nydrazid, INH, Niadox)	Increased phenytoin toxicity
Methotrexate	Salicylates	Increased methotrexate effects and toxicity of methotrexate

Sources: The Medical Letter, vol. 17, Feb. 28, 1975; Patient Care (special section), Dec. 1, 1974, pp. 172–174; Current Prescribing (Anticoagulants), June 1976, pp. 42–66; Drug Therapy (Antihypertensive Drug Reactions), Dec. 1974, pp. 49–55; Emergency Medicine (Drug + Drug), Dec. 1971, pp. 21–34. Table prepared by Lederle Laboratories, A Division of American Cynamid Company.

Chapter 6

Gastrointestinal Drugs

LAXATIVES

It is appropriate to start a discussion of gastrointestinal drugs with laxatives. They are the most overused and abused of all drugs, if for no other reason than that they can be bought and used without a prescription. Commerce in laxatives probably amounts to hundreds of millions of dollars. Advertising of laxatives is all-pervasive. Radio and television, newspapers, magazines, billboards, and word of mouth all lead many people to believe that laxatives are necessary to a healthy life. Hundreds of thousands, if not millions, of people have adopted laxative lore as a matter of faith. For many people the use of laxatives has been a lifelong custom, passed on from generation to generation.

It is little wonder, then, that a bulky, easy bowel movement becomes a libidinal desire for many old people. In their youth they may have been given calomel or Crazy Crystals, violent purges that were supposed to excrete poisons from the systems. (Calomel, a mercury-containing compound, has long since been outlawed. Crazy Crystals, sodium sulfate, has an action like Epsom salt.)

Given the kind of laxative indoctrination we have been talking about, the symptom of constipation is of great concern in old people. On the average, old people are less active physically. They probably eat less. Most old people don't get enough fiber in their diet. They may take constipating drugs. With impaired thirst sensations they are apt to drink too little liquid. The fecal urge may be less sensitive. Isolation and depression cause people to become self–conscious.

In light of the general knowledge that bowel symptoms are often due to serious disease, it is little wonder that bowel preoccupation asserts itself. We wish to emphasize, though, that the preoccupation is frequently more severe and stubborn, and more difficult to treat rationally, than organic disease.

Only a few years ago, fiber-free diets were prescribed for almost any digestive ailment ranging from poor teeth to hermorrhoids. "Too much roughage" was thought harmful for stomach ulcers or diverticulosis of the colon. Consequently, many old people shun fruits, cereals, and vegetables, which are conducive to the kind of bowel action most of them crave.

Milk, aside from being nutritious, has been assigned some mysterious health-giving role. As a matter of fact, about 25 percent of old people don't tolerate milk very well. A deficiency of lactase, a digestive enzyme, may cause many old people to have cramps, flatus, and diarrhea. These symptoms of milk intolerance can cause some old people to take laxatives or, more often, a constipating anticholinergic agent.

Sometimes people take laxatives to "break the laxative habit," thus substituting one for another. We shall talk about placebos in a later chapter, but the placebo effect is present in the color, the physical appearance, and the advertising of nearly all medicines, especially laxatives.

When speaking of laxative use and abuse, it should be pointed out that they have very few legitimate medical uses. One of the few uses is to clear the bowel for certain x-ray examinations and in preparation for surgery. Sufficient water, bulk, and fiber in the diet and sufficient exercise are enough to promote bowel action in a healthy person.

Laxatives may become necessary if a person eats poorly, drinks poorly, doesn't exercise enough, takes a constipating medicine, or, rarely, has a particular disease of the bowel. More often than not, however, if a bowel is diseased, laxatives should be avoided.

Among the reasons laxatives are used so much is that they rarely do truly serious harm. Grandparents may go for years without developing severe symptoms from using their favorite laxatives. When they become old and feeble, however, there is a greater risk. Fluid and electrolyte loss through the bowel can and often does aggravate a number of other problems, most often undiagnosed. For example, if an old person is taking a digitalis preparation for heart trouble in addition to a laxative the loss of potassium through the gut can subject him or her to the chance of serious complications that may not be blamed at all upon the laxative.

Now let's be more technical. Constipation is caused by a variety of factors in the aging gut, including muscle atrophy, thickened mucous membranes, a blander diet, less physical activity, and a blunting of visceral sensations. Adding to all this are such commonly used constipating drugs as anticholinergics, antidepressants, antispasmodics, narcotics, propoxyphene (Darvon), phenothiazines, antihypertensives such as hydralazine (Apresoline), some antacids, and, paradoxically, a reliance on laxatives.

Laxatives can be grouped by their general methods of action:

1 *Stimulant* Laxatives cause increased peristalsis in the colon. There are two major subgroups: (1) anthraquinones, such as casanthranol, cascara, senna, and danthron and (2) diphenylmethanes, which include bisacodyl and phenolphthalein. Bisacodyl, which can be taken orally or as a suppository, is an effective agent which has no known systemic effects. Phenolphthalein is cyclically absorbed, excreted in the bile, and reabsorbed and thus may act for several days to produce a watery stool. Its excessive use can cause fluid and electrolyte imbalances, and large doses can cause diarrhea, cardiac and respiratory distress, and various skin eruptions. Because many elderly persons have decreased fluid and electrolyte reserves as well as various cardiac difficulties, the regular use of pheonolphthalein laxatives should be avoided if possible. The prolonged use of stimulant laxatives can lead to disappearance of nerve cells in the colon resulting in denervation, to atrophy of the smooth muscle coat, and to pigmentation of the colon.

2 *Saline* laxatives act osmotically in both the large and small intestines to draw in fluid, thus increasing pressure in the bowel lumen. The added pressure, in turn, stimulates peristalsis. They are usually either magnesium or sodium phosphate salts. A significant amount of magnesium may be absorbed but is so quickly excreted by the kidneys that an increased level is rarely found in the blood. However, if there is inadequate kidney function, magnesium may accumulate. Declining renal function with age is discussed in a previous chapter under pharmacokinetc considerations. Large quantities of sodium salts can be hazardous to those on low-sodium diets and in congestive heart failure. The action of all these osmotically acting drugs starts in the small intestine, where the intestinal contents are semiliquid. Large doses cause a watery diarrhea which, in turn, may lead to fluid and electrolyte imbalance or depletion.

3 *Stool softeners* such as dioctyl sodium sulfosuccinate and dioctyl calcium sulfosuccinate act by helping water to penetrate and soften hard, dry stools, and thus ease passage of such stools through the colon. They are sometimes combined with stimulant laxatives. To be fully effective it is essential for the patient to drink enough fluid. There is a nutritional consideration with these stool softeners. Dioctyl sodium sulfosuccinate reduces the digestive capacity of the gastric juice on dietary proteins at a concentration well below that used in laxative therapy. It decreases the volume of stomach secretions and has a direct inhibitory effect on pepsin.

4 *Lubricants* coat and soften the fecal mass and smooth its passage along the intestines. The most commonly used lubricant is mineral oil. The chronic use of mineral oil can cause a variety of problems. In those persons with such predisposing factors as debility, senility, and faulty swallowing mechanisms, lipoid pneumonia may arise from the chronic use of mineral oil. A small amount remaining in the pharynx from a bedtime dose may seep into the bronchioles where it accumulates and causes inflammation and fibrosis, leading to decreased

maximal breathing capacity and decreased arterial oxygen saturation. Then compensatory respiratory acidosis and decreased pulmonary capacity may ensue. Mineral oil may be absorbed, especially when given with wetting or emulsifying agents such as dioctyl sodium sulfosuccinate. It then becomes localized in mesenteric lymph nodes, the intestinal mucosa, the liver, and the spleen, impairing the function of these organs. The absorption of calcium, phosphate, and vitamins A and D may be decreased. Large doses passing through the anal sphincter may cause pruritis, hemorrhoids, and related anal problems.

5 *Bulk laxatives* generally include such products as psyllium seed colloids or cellulose derivatives, often with dextrose. They are represented by such products as Metamucil, Mucilose, Siblin, and Serutan. They form bulky gels in the intestines to stimulate peristalsis. They are not absorbed and do not seem to have any particular side effects. They should be taken with plenty of water and should be avoided when there seems to be intestinal obstruction or impaction. Some contain up to 50 percent dextrose, which may be a consideration for those on diabetic diets. They may combine with and decrease the absorption and activity of salicylates and digitalis drugs.

ANTACIDS

We shall now discuss antacids, also highly advertised and generally available without prescription. Their use is not as harmless as most people believe, and their use may delay accurate diagnosis of a serious condition.

All antacid products contain one or more of the following ingredients—aluminum oxide, hydroxide, or phosphate; calcium carbonate; magnesium oxide, carbonate, or trisilicate; sodium or potassium bicarbonate; dihydroxyaluminum acetate or aminoacetate; or bismuth subnitrate. Others may contain proteins, milk solids, simethicone, or aromatic oils. When selecting an antacid, the person should consider at least the following factors: (1) cost versus neutralizing capacity, (2) other effects of the antacid, and (3) sodium content.

Most antacids decrease the absorption of anticoagulants, barbiturates, lithium, methenamine, nalidixic acid, nitrofurantoin, penicillin, salicylates, tetracycline, chlorpromazine, digitalis drugs, and ampicillin. They increase the absorption of allopurinol, amitriptyline, quinidine, and anticholinergics. What can these antacids do in addition to neutralizing stomach acid? Many things. Routine doses of sodium bicarbonate may be large enough to lead to systemic alkalosis and sodium retention, especially if renal function is declining. They may also cause an acid rebound.

A fair amount of calcium may be absorbed from the stomach. Several days of use of calcium-containing antacids may lead to hypercalcemia and its attendant neurological problems and renal calculi and decreased renal function. In addition, calcium salts induce the secretion of additional acid, and they may also be constipating. Although intermittent low doses may be safe, they cause too many severe and frequent side effects for continuous treatment.

Aluminum salts are also constipating, especially in elderly persons. To counteract this, many are combined with magnesium salts, which have a laxative action. Aluminum was implicated as a possible causative agent in neurological syndromes and dementia when chronic users had elevated aluminum levels in their brains. However, elevated aluminum levels may also be due to declining renal excretion. The subject of aluminum in dementia will be discussed under chronic brain syndromes and Alzheimer's disease in Chapter 9. Also of importance to the elderly person is the effect of aluminum on phosphate. As a result of the formation of aluminum phosphate in the intestines, serum levels of phosphate may decline, leading to loss of calcium phosphate from bones. In turn, this leads to osteomalacia, often in as little as 3 weeks after starting therapy.

Antacids are often taken for such symptoms as heartburn, gas, belching, and regurgitation, all of which occur frequently in elderly people. Such symptoms are not necessarily associated with hyperacidity, especially since stomach acid tends to diminish with age. Most antacids have a demulcent, or coating, action that relieves some of the above symptoms, regardless of their acid-neutralizing effects. Indeed, there is doubt whether antacids are of value in treating peptic ulcers. Their use leads to greater secretion of acid through the rebound phenomenon, i.e., enhanced acid secretion resulting from a temporary lowering of stomach acidity.

As with any other drug, an occasional dose of an antacid for some minor GI problem is of no great consequence. However, its long-term use for undiagnosed GI distress is not so innocuous since it may result in unnecessary delays in proper diagnosis of more serious problems such as ulcers, cancer, and diverticulitis. The pharmacist should verify with the customer that the problem is minor and is not one that has persisted for weeks or months. While working in a small community pharmacy in Michigan we talked with many patrons who came in for antacids. Many had problems which had started months previously, but had not considered them serious enough to seek medical attention. These people were advised to see their doctors.

Regardless of purely scientific or theoretical considerations, however, millions of people take many millions of doses of antacids. We are not prepared to argue that some of them are not relieved of their symptoms, at least temporarily. We are prepared to say, though, that antacids should not be taken continually or indiscriminately. In particular, they should not be used often without at least looking for potentially serious disease.

Assuming one is going to use an antacid often, which preparation should one use? The graphic demonstration of antacid action one sees on television could lead one to assume that most of us humans are in a life-or-death struggle against acidity. If so, we should use the most effective, least expensive, and least harmful antacid we can get. Table 6-1 lists the most frequently used antacids. Generally, it is wise for old people to use those with lower sodium content.

ANTICHOLINERGICS

We talked at length about anticholinergic drugs in Chapter 4. They are used mainly in treating gastrointestinal symptoms such as diarrhea and spasm that may

Table 6-1 Most Frequently Used Antacids

Antacid	Milliequivalents acid neutralized by 1 mL antacid	Volume of antacid required to neutralize 100 meq HCl	Milligrams of sodium in amount sufficient to neutralize 100 meq HCl	Wholesale cost *per 12 oz †per pint ‡tablets	Wholesale cost per 100 meq acid neutralized
Mylanta II	4.14	24.1	20–48	$2.57*	$0.17
Titralac	3.87	25.9	57	1.80*	0.13
Camalox	3.59	27.9	14	2.40†	0.14
Aludrox	2.81	35.6	10.7	1.83*	0.11
Maalox	2.58	38.7	19	1.73*	0.19
Creamalin	2.57	38.9	?	2.60†	0.21
Di-Gel	2.45	40.9	70	1.60*	0.18
Mylanta	2.38	42	33	1.66*	0.19
Silain-Gel	2.31	43.3	41.6	1.60*	0.19
Riopan	2.21	45.3	6.3	1.50*	0.19
Amphogel	1.93	51.9	72	1.83*	0.26
Kolantyl gel	1.69	59.1	?	1.50*	0.25
Gelusil	1.33	75.3	120	1.53*	0.32
Phosphalgel	0.42	238.1	595	1.65*	1.09
Milk of Magnesia Phillips	2.8	35.7	?	1.04*	0.10
Phillips-Roxane				0.62*	0.06
Tums	5.5 meq/tablet	18 tablets	49		
Alka-Seltzer	4 meq/tablet	25 tablets	6900	2.40/72‡	0.83

manifest themselves in cramps and pain. Simply put, the anticholinergics are used to quiet the gut, i.e., to reduce gastrointestinal motility and secretion. They are useful in treating such diverse organic diseases as colitis, peptic ulcer, and diverticulitis. They can help in such purely functional or nervous conditions as spastic colon or nervous indigestion.

The naturally occurring anticholinergics are atropine, belladonna, and scopolamine. A large number of synthetic and semisynthetic compounds have actions which vary only slightly from the natural compounds. They are sold by different manufacturers under the names Banthine, Bentyl, Cantil, Daricon, Lomotil, Pamine, Probanthine, Robinul, Valpin, and many more. All manufacturers promote their own products as having special merit or being more or less effective for a certain action. All undoubtedly could adduce evidence that their products are superior in on way or another, but we remain skeptical of such claims.

As expected from previous discussion, anticholinergics reduce gastrointestinal motility and secretion. They dry the mouth. They are apt to cause constipation and are therefore useful in diarrhea. They tend to relieve bladder spasm as well as gastrointestinal spasm; therefore, they are useful in relieving urinary burning and frequency. They all have a tendency to dilate the pupils and are thus dangerous to use in people with glaucoma. (Glaucoma is an eye condition often leading to blindness and is one of the few conditions treated with cholinergic drugs, which constrict the pupils, thereby relieving the dangerous pressure in the eyeballs.)

Let us consider some of the very serious things that may happen when a person uses an anticholingergic drug. An elderly man with, say, a peptic ulcer goes to his doctor. The doctor may order the standard treatment for peptic ulcer, an antacid and an anticholinergic. The medicines almost immediately enable the old man to forget his burning stomach. Instead, his vision blurs and he cannot read his newspaper. He may develop severe eye pain and redness, which his eye doctor diagnoses as glaucoma. His mouth becomes dry, his speech becomes slurred, and his dentures don't fit. (If he still has his own teeth, he may develop irritation of his gums from the protracted dryness of his mouth.) The old gentleman most likely will become constipated and take a laxative, undoing to an extent the effects of the anticholinergic. It is likely that he will begin to have difficulty in urinating; his stream may be reduced to a dribble or cut off entirely.

We do not wish to imply that anticholinergics are dangerous most of the time in most people. We do wish to say that among the old, reactions to them are common and occasionally severe.

It is appropriate here to state that many psychotropic drugs and a number of drugs used for Parkinson's disease have anticholinergic effects. These drugs will be discussed later.

A relatively new gastrointestinal drug should probably be mentioned here before we go on to another chapter. It is cimetidine, trade named Tagamet. It is a promising drug in the treatment of gastric acidity and peptic ulcer. We have had no experience with it, but it is not an acid neutralizer or an anticholinergic. Instead, it works directly on the parietal cells of the stomach to inhibit acid secretion. So far, it appears it will be useful in treating hyperacidity and in reducing the use of antacids and anticholinergics.

We go now to cardiovascular drugs.

Chapter 7

Drugs Used in Cardiovascular Disease

More people die of heart and blood vessel disease than of any other cause. High blood pressure, excessive fatty substances in the blood, and diabetes all predispose to cardiovascular disease. Strokes, heart attacks, and impaired circulation in the legs or other parts of the body are seen frequently in a geriatrics practice.

The underlying condition in most cardiovascular disease of old people is arteriosclerosis, or more particularly *atherosclerosis*, in which aggregates of fatty substances are deposited in blood-vessel linings. Blood clots are apt to form about these deposits, thus decreasing or shutting off blood flow. (Figure 7-1)

If a clot forms in a coronary artery the process is called *coronary thrombosis*, and the victim is said to have had a heart attack. If a clot forms in one of the vessels supplying blood to the brain, the victim may develop any number of symptoms, among them paralysis, and is said to have had a stroke. If a clot shuts off the supply to a sufficiently large part of a limb, that part will undergo gangrene.

It is not necessary to have blood clots and atherosclerosis, though, to have heart trouble or dementia. High blood pressure alone puts a burden on the heart. In certain states of poor nutrition or advanced age, hearts and brains may fail. Indeed, atherosclerosis and blood clots are not responsible for most cases of

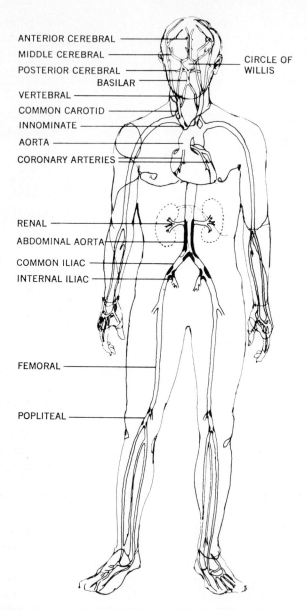

Figure 7-1   Common sites for atherosclerotic lesions. (*From Fill and File 58(4):60 (1972), published by Eli Lilly and Company, Indianapolis, Indiana..*)

congestive heart failure or senile dementia. *Hardening of the arteries* is a lay term widely accepted as being responsible for many ills, and for this the geriatrician can be grateful. Such a term is an imprecise appellation for the inscrutable, unavoidable, inexorable processes that affect old people.

Later, we shall discuss digitalis drugs. The chief use of these drugs is in congestive heart failure. Congestive heart failure is a result of the heart's inability to pump enough blood to meet the demands put upon it. When the heart is unable to pump the blood presented to it, the blood collects in the lungs, causing congestion. The patient with congestion in the lungs due to a failing heart is said to have congestive heart failure.

Among the causes of congestive heart failure is hypertension. In most instances the cause of hypertension is not known. It affects men more than women and blacks more than whites. Hypertension puts a burden on the heart and predisposes to stroke and impaired kidney function. Victims of high blood pressure either improve or suffer from serious illness or death before they grow old. For reasons that will be pointed out, it is seldom wise to initiate treatment for hypertension in old people. Systolic blood pressure is the pressure when the heart is in systole, the state of cardiac contraction. Diastolic blood pressure is measured during diastole, when the heart is relaxed.

Now let's proceed to a more technical discussion. From age 20 to 65, arterial systolic blood pressure increases 17 percent in males and 24 percent in females. The rise stops after 65 in men and 75 in women, and there is then a gradual decline. Diastolic pressure rises until age 40, then fails to keep up with systolic rise and declines after age 65. Venous pressure shows no change or correlation with age and is not significantly altered.

Benign arterial hypertension is generally associated with the natural changes of aging. There is a gradual increase in irritability of the vasoconstrictor medullary center in the brain produced by minute ischemic arteriosclerotic lesions or by deterioration of specific neuron groups within the area, thus leading to a vaso-pressor response.

Caution should be exercised in initiating drug therapy for hypertension in the older patient because of the greater incidence of cornonary insufficiency, arteriosclerosis, and renal impairment. The drugs of choice are those with a mild persistent action such as the thiazides.

It is unlikely that drugs can reduce arteriosclerotic-induced hypertension, which is characterized by high systolic and nearly normal diastolic pressure, as the vessel walls are inelastic and less responsive. However, if a large enough dose is given so as to alter homeostatic mechanisms stabilizing blood pressure, there may be disastrous consequences. Hypotension, reduced cardiac output, and cerebral and coronary insufficiency may result, with little improvement in the hypertension. Less serious effects include dizziness, palpitations, increased angina, and fatigue. In true hypertension, where diastolic pressure is elevated, lack of treatment may lead to cardiac insufficiency and a further reduction of cardiac reserve.

Severe blood pressure reduction may seriously impair glomerular filtration, and renal function should be regularly evaluated to prevent azotemia or uremia.

Cerebrovascular disease of any severity is usually a contraindication to the energetic treatment of hypertension in the elderly as lowering the blood pressure may hasten mental deterioration. In the healthy 70-year-old male, cerebral blood pressure and vascular resistance have increased and cerebral blood flow has decreased by 7 percent since age 21. Decreases greater than this are attributed to arteriosclerosis and not to age per se.

Although coronary blood flow decreases with age, the decrease is less than the decrease in cardiac output, so in the healthy individual relative coronary flow changes little with age, but is decreased with coronary disease.

We shall proceed to a brief discussion of several agents used in the treatment of hypertension:

Antihypertension Therapy

Rauwolfia Products   The frequency of side reactions to rauwolfia products limits their use mainly to mild hypertension. Less serotonin in the aging brain may account for the doubled incidence of mental depression, often of the agitated type following the use of rauwolfia products in the elderly. The sedation by rauwolfia may also mask various types of cerebral dysfunction. An unsteady gait and a Parkinson-like syndrome, discussed later, occur frequently when rauwoulfia products are used by older people and may threaten their emotional stability and ability to care for themselves.

Vagal stimulation by rauwolfia may cause atrial slowing in the patient taking digitalis. Unless the physician realizes that the bradycardia is caused by the rauwolfia, digitalis dosage may be reduced, to the harm of the patient.

The elderly person on rauwolfia undergoing surgery presents a real problem. Anesthesia aggravates the hypotensive effect of the drug. With an abrupt fall in blood pressure, coronary thrombosis, cerebral thrombosis, or kidney failure are much more likely. This kind of emergency can arise with other antihypertensives as well as with a number of psychotropic drugs, which we will discuss later.

Ganglionic Blockers   These should rarely if ever be used in older persons. They may enhance a preexisting orthostatic hypotension seen in elderly hypertensive patients, who may faint if blood pressure falls abruptly when they stand. These patients should be advised to rise slowly and avoid prolonged motionless standing.

An acute cerebral vascular episode may follow the use of ganglionic blockers and is characterized by apathy, confusion, disorientation, and a shocklike pallor and clammy skin for as long as three to four hours after administration of the drug.

Injudicious use of ganglionic blockers in patients with diverticulosis can precipitate constipation, obstipation, and paralytic ileus.

Hydralazine (Apresoline)   This drug works principally by relaxing smooth muscle cells in the walls of small arteries. It increases heart rate, work, and output and may lead to coronary insufficiency. Long-term use indicates that lowering the blood pressure with hydralazine does not prevent further cardiac deterioration in the elderly. Contraindications to hydralazine, as with any hypotensive agent, include congestive heart failure, severe coronary artery disease, severe cerebral disease, or advanced renal insufficiency. These contraindications preclude its use in old people except in the most unusual circumstances.

Beta-Adrenergic Inhibitors In Chapter 4, we mentioned that antiadrenergic agents had limited but important uses. We were thinking then of propranolol, a beta-adrenergic blocking agent. A word here about definitions:

> On the basis of differences in pharmacologic activity of similarly structured catecholamines, investigators originally postulated that the activity of the adrenergic (sympathetic) portion of the human autonomic nervous system is mediated by stimulation of two types of receptors: alpha and beta. The alpha (α) receptors are found predominantly in the blood vessels of the skin, mucosa, intestine, and kidney and their stimulation results in vasoconstrition in these vascular beds. The beta (β) receptors predominate in the heart, the arteries and arterioles of skeletal muscle, and in the bronchi of the lungs. Stimulation of these results in cardiac excitation, vasodilation, and bronchodilation.
>
> Subsequent investigation has provided evidence for the existence of two types of beta receptors, designated as beta$_1$ and beta$_2$ receptors. For the purpose of this disussion, the beta$_2$ receptors primarily mediate the beta-adrenergic effects on the heart while the beta$_2$ receptors mediate the effects on the lungs and peripheral muscles. Although no receptors have ever been identified anatomically, these concepts have been accepted as a physiologic model to explain the pharmacologic actions of various adrenergic agonists (stimulators) and antagonists (blockers).[1]

Propranolol, then, is useful in a number of ways. It is helpful in the treatment of certain irregularities of heartbeat. It may be useful in hypertension and in angina pectoris, a painful condition usually caused by an insufficiency of blood flow through the coronary arteries.

Unfortunately, propranolol may precipitate congestive heart failure in a patient with an impaired heart muscle. In a susceptible person, life-threatening asthma may be induced by this very useful drug. The drug should not be stopped abruptly, for doing so has resulted in life-threatening irregularities of the heartbeat and in coronary thrombosis.

Diuretics In some way not fully understood, salt depletion reduces blood pressure, perhaps by reducing the amount of body fluids. Regardless of the exact mechanisms, thiazide diuretics have been a blessing to many people with high blood pressure. There are as many as twenty of these or related drugs sold under different trade names but with only slightly different modes of action. They act upon the kidneys to enhance the excretion of water, salt, and potassium. In addition to their use in high blood pressure, diuretics are useful in congestive heart failure, in which excess fluid accumulates in lungs, limbs, and elsewhere.

Generally, thiazide diuretics are safe when their use is adequately monitored. They may cause potassium depletion, and for this reason some of our medical colleagues routinely prescribe a potassium salt in one of its several forms. In old people potassium medication with its attendant nuisance, expense, unpleasant taste, and occasional toxicity can be avoided by proper attention to diet. Fruits, fruit juices, coffee, and most vegetables are rich in potassium. This is not to say that potassium depletion may not on occasion be serious. It may enhance the tendency toward digitalis toxicity and may cause cardiac arrhythmias and general muscle weakness.

Far more frequent than potassium depletion is water depletion, i.e., dehydration, which is particularly apt to occur in old people, whose sense of thirst is likely to be impaired. Not infrequently, we have been called to treat a weak, slightly confused old person when the nurse reports that he or she is ''just not doing well today.'' We find that the mouth is dry and the skin is inelastic and lacks its usual turgor. On checking, we find that the patient takes a diuretic for heart failure and has become depleted of water. The treatment is, of course, to give extra fluid by mouth or through a needle, depending on the urgency of the matter.

While discussing diuretics, furosemide (Lasix) should be mentioned. It has the same general actions as thiazides, although its diuretic action is more pronounced dose for dose. In general, it is used more for edema and congestive heart failure than for high blood pressure. Generally, it requires the same type of monitoring as the thiazides.

Methyldopa (Aldomet)   The action of this drug is not fully understood. Apparently it works on the central nervous system to inhibit the production of adrenergic substances. It may cause excessive sedation or depression in an old person. It may cause postural hypotension with resulting faintness. Occasionally, it will cause salt and water retention with edema. Like many other drugs, it has, on rare occasions, caused fever, liver damage, and anemia. Unlike ganglionic blockers, it is relatively safe to use in old people if closely monitored.

Digitalis Therapy

Four main factors predispose the elderly to digitalis intoxication:

1   Slower excretion prolongs the half-life of the drug. The increase is from about 51 hours in young subjects to about 73 hours in the old. Equal doses in young and old can produce twice the blood level in the older persons because of changes in body composition resulting in a different volume of distribution.

2   The vagus is particularly sensitive in older persons, and digitalization may result in bradycardia sufficient to cause dizziness and partial or complete heart block.

3   Diuretic therapy or laxative abuse can induce hypokalemia, increasing the heart's sensitivity to digitalis.

4 Control with longer-acting preparations such as digitoxin (as compared with digoxin) may be more difficult. An asymptomatic digitalis toxicity is more likely to develop.

Here are four examples of adverse reactions to digitalis commonly seen in the elderly:

1 There may be anorexia instead of nausea and vomiting, as in the case of Mrs. O. (Chapter 3).

2 Muddy or hazy vision and white or yellow halos may be seen about bright objects instead of changes in color vision.

3 There may be arrhythmias without other signs of toxicity.

4 Common central nervous system signs of toxicity include malaise, mental confusion, and depression.

Digitalis-induced gynecomastia has been found in older men. Their relative lack of androgens enhances the estrogenic activity of the digitalis aglycone. There are at least three causes of digitalis failure in the aged.

1 Long-standing heart disease may have reduced cardiac reserve too far for any real improvement.

2 Peripheral oxygen demand may be increased rather than cardiac output functionally reduced. For example thyrotoxicosis, frequently masked in the aged, may be manifested in congestive heart failure, which reflects an increased cellular metabolism and excessive demand on an arteriosclerotic heart.

3 Decreased oxygen transport capacity as in anemia may cause excessive demand on the heart's pumping ability.

Requirements for digitalis decrease with age, and it is important that aged persons on digitalis be evaluated periodically to determine whether the drug should be continued. A careful evaluation of a geriatric population may find that in nearly half, digitalis may be discontinued. Digitalis may have been started when an acute illness increased the heart burden and caused myocardial insufficiency, but was not stopped when the complicating condition cleared. Much digitalis therapy for heart failure may have been initiated under questionable or doubtful circumstances, without good documentation of cardiac failure. Complaints of decreased appetite, listlessness, and being withdrawn and quarrelsome may decrease when digitalis is withdrawn.

Vasodilator Therapy

Vasodilator drugs are used to increase the perfusion of blood in parts where blood flow may be impaired. Nicotinic acid, one of the B vitamins, in a sufficently large dose will cause vasodilatation and flushing of the skin. Several times we have seen old people frightened and flushed with an uncomfortable warmth of the skin and pounding in the head. They had taken their dose of nicotinic acid "for the circulation" on an empty stomach, thus ensuring its rapid absorption in quantity sufficient to cause frightening symptoms which they thought were due to strokes or heart attacks.

Unfortunately, the possible benefits of certain other vasodilators, some of which contain nicotinic acid, are just as doubtful. Yet they are often prescribed for symptoms ranging from dizzy spells to gangrene of the feet. Though it may seem otherwise, we are not in the denouncing business. We believe, though, that most vasodilators are useful only for their placebo effects.

The outstanding exception is the nitrites, used in angina pectoris, always a potentially serious malady. It is caused by an absolute or relative insufficiency of oxygen to the heart muscle. Angina pectoris is frequently a precursor of coronary thrombosis, though it may be present for years without serious complication. It is most often due to atherosclerosis of one or more of the coronary arteries. When patients with coronary sclerosis become excited or exert themselves excessively, the need of the heart muscle for oxygen is increased. Since narrowed vessels cannot carry an increased flow of blood, pain warns the patient to relax and slow down.

Nitrites can dilate the coronary vessels promptly, thus reducing the danger and the pain. There are long-acting and short-acting nitrites. Nitroglycerin is the best known coronary vasodilator and perhaps the most reliable. There are no serious complications resulting from its use but it may cause flushing, a pounding headache, a prickly sensation, or faintness.

Organic nitrates are frequently prescribed for impaired coronary circulation. They work by being converted to nitrites. Their benefit is often unpredictable or uncertain because they are in large measure degraded in the liver, and, thus, not much of the drug reaches the general circulation.

Anticoagulant Therapy

Old people are particularly vulnerable to *thrombosis*, the clotting of blood in situ, and *embolism*, the dislodging of a clot to a distant site. Thus we often hear of blood clots in the brain, i.e. *cerebral thrombosis* or in the coronary arteries, *coronary thrombosis*. Thrombophlebitis is a troublesome condition, usually occurring in the legs, whose chief danger is that clots will be dislodged to become lodged in the lung, leading to *pulmonary embolism*.

In the late forties researchers found that warfarin, derived originally from sweet clover, would reduce the clotting tendency and enhance the bleeding tendency of blood. At first, warfarin and its chemical descendents were considered a great boon to people who were in danger of clotting complications. They remain useful in several branches of medicine. Perhaps no medicine requires closer monitoring with laboratory tests, is so subject to interference by other drugs, or can be more disastrous in its untoward effects.

Our experience is that anticoagulants are often prescribed unwisely for long-term use since they function chiefly as very dangerous placebos. We believe they should be used in a hospital with monitoring by experienced laboratory and nursing personnel. We deplore their use in confused old people who may be taking other drugs. Serious hemorrhage or a sense of misguided security occurs too often with long-term use of anticoagulants in old people.

SUMMARY

We have discussed the drugs used most frequently in cardiovascular disease. Several others deserve mention. Quinidine is frequently used to help regulate faulty heart rhythm. It may cause ringing in the ears, giddiness, faintness, nausea, and diarrhea. Its use is often unpredictable and it should not be prescribed without clear indications and close monitoring. Clonidine may produce drowsiness and impotence. Since it is a relatively new drug, we don't believe its use in old people is justified at this time.

In a book like this we should at least mention cholesterol, a fatty substance in the blood that plays a role in the clogging of arteries. Most people with marked elevation of cholesterol do not live to be geriatric patients. We have not had occasion to treat elevated cholesterol, although several drugs, combined with marked diet restriction, are said to be useful. In our elderly patients we occasionally suggest a diet low in saturated fat if the cholesterol is elevated.

We have given our views on most of the commonly used drugs in old people with cardiovascular disease. Again, we say that more good than harm will be done by prescribing the very minimum of the very fewest. Among old people it is remarkable how well many get along with no medicine at all.

We now direct our attention to drugs that work upon the central nervous system.

REFERENCES

1 P. H. Vlasser, "Beta-blockers: An Update," *Guidelines to Professional Pharmacy,* **3**(4)(1977).

Chapter 8

Mind Drugs

The most frequently prescribed drugs are those that affect mood or conscious-ness. As a group they have been both a blessing and a curse. They have enabled mental hospitals to close or decrease their number of beds. They have enabled disabled people to return to their families and to the workaday world. At the same time they have engendered the notion that many day-to-day stresses are unendur-able and thus require medication. In turn, an illicit commerce has been promoted, addiction has become commonplace, and innocent people have been victimized by an unwise reliance on drugs.

Old people are no exception to the above generalization. They are, how-ever, more susceptible to undesireable drug reactions for a number of reasons. Retirement, ill health, grief, reduced social status, diminished income, hospital-ization, institutionalization, and other unfortunate circumstances are more upset-ting on the average to an elderly person than to a younger person. An older person is more apt to be taking a drug incompatible with a mind drug. Old people are much more subject to pathological depression than young people. Therefore, old people may require more medication for life-related stress at a time when their minds and bodies are least able to handle such chemical manipulation.

The aging central nervous system is quite sensitive to mind drugs for several reasons:

1 Decreasing numbers of nerve cells result in stimulants being less effective and depressants more potent; the individual's pharmacokinetics change for reasons discussed earlier.

2 The number of potentially interacting drugs is greater in the old than the young.

3 Cerebral blood flow is reduced, especially in those with cerebral arteriosclerosis.

All brain areas are not equally affected. The rate of neuron loss varies in different phylogenetic areas. The unequal loss upsets the balance of interactions among the various cerebral centers. Integrated brain function deteriorates, providing a mechanism for altered reactivity and sensitivity. Thus the older person may show paradoxical and unusual reactions to drugs.

Since psychotropic drugs are so important, the following outline may be useful:

Minor tranquilizers (antianxiety)
Barbiturates: phenobarbital, butabarbital, amobarbital
Propanediols: meprobamate, tybamate
Benzodiazepines: chlordiazepoxide (Librium), chlorazepate (Tranxene), diazepam (Valium), oxazepam (Serax)
Sedating antihistamines: hydroxyzine (Atarax, Vistaril), promethazine (Phenergan)

Hypnotics
Glutethimide (Doriden), chloral hydrate, barbiturates, etchlorvynol (Placidyl), flurazepam (Dalmane), benzodiazepine

Major tranquilizers (antipsychotics)
Phenothiazines
Dimethylaminopropyl derivatives: chlorpromazine (Thorazine), promazine (Sparine), promethazine (Phenergan)
Piperidine derivatives: mesoridazine (Serentil), piperacetazine (Quide), thioridazine (Mellaril)
Piperazine derivatives: fluphenazine (Permitil, Prolixin), perphenazine (Trilafon), prochlorperazine (Compazine), trifluoperazine (Stelazine)
Butyrophenones: haloperidol (Haldol)
Thioxanthenes
Dimethylaminopropyl derivatives: chlorprothixene (Taractan)
Piperazine derivatives: thiothixene (Navane)

Antidepressants
Monoamine oxidase inhibitors: isocarboxizid (Marplan), phenelzine (Nardil), tranylcypromine (Parnate)
Tricyclic Antidepressants
Dibenzazepines: imipramine (Tofranil, Presamine) and desipramine (Norpramin, Pertofrane)

Dibenzocycloheptenes: amitriptyline (Elavil), nortriptyline (Aventyl), protriptyline (Vivactyl)
Dibenzoxepine: doxepin (Sinequan, Adapin)

MINOR TRANQUILIZERS

Benzodiazepines do not seem to induce the despair or depression sometimes seen with phenothiazines and meprobamate. Older patients generally require smaller doses than young adults. Relatively small doses of diazepam have induced stuporousness, sluggishness, drowsiness, and impaired gait when used in a variety of geriatric psychiatric illnesses, although these effects will usually clear with a smaller dose. Because benzodiazepines are relatively mild drugs; are widely used for mild nervousness, anxiety, and other vague complaints, and are relatively expensive, it is interesting to compare them to placebos in men from 60 to 75 years and 75 years and over. Diazepam produced small but significant decreases in depression, but also decreased memory, intellectual function, and motor function, and increased fatigue, especially in the older men. The antianxiety effects of diazepam are generally limited to younger people. The older men had more consistent reduction in anxiety from placebos, which, of course, had no sedative or depressing effects. The placebos in the older men, surprisingly, reduced fatigue and improved memory and motor function.

HYPNOTICS (SLEEPING MEDICATIONS)

A common complaint by aging persons is their inability to sleep. Their insomnia may be caused by depression, pain, tension, nocturia, muscle cramps, or overuse of caffeine. However, much geriatric "insomnia" represents a normal reduction in sleep requirements with age. While the young adult may need 7 to 8 hours of sleep a night, the old person may need only 4⅛ to 6⅛ hours.

Since sleep disorders are so common, a brief discussion is warranted. There are two basic kinds of sleep: (1) REM (rapid eye movement) sleep, which occupies about 25 percent of sleeping time and is the stage where dreaming occurs, and (2) non-REM sleep, which occupies the remaining 75 percent and is divided into four stages: from stage 1, which is light dozing, to stage 4, which is deep sleep. In non-REM sleep, there is little mental or physical activity, and it is here that sleep disturbances occur. Aging is associated with a sharp reduction in stage 3 and stage 4, so that the feeling of deep sleep is missing. The person may complain of never sleeping, even though all-night EEG monitors show that the person spent hours in stage 1 and stage 2.

Most sleeping preparations are successful for a short time, and it is easier to impose a synthetic sleep than to diagnose the cause of insomnia or assure the patient. While an occasional sedative may be justified, chronic use rarely is and may lead quickly to dependence. Barbiturates, glutethimide, and methyprylon (Noludar) significantly reduce REM sleep; this is followed by REM breakthrough, drug efficacy is diminished, and the dose is increased. If the drug is discontinued, there may be REM rebound with nightmares, insomnia, and disordered sleep. Chronic insomniacs on hypnotics often have a more difficult time sleeping than unmedicated insomniacs. In contrast, flurazepam (Dalmane) produces only minor REM suppression, no rebound, and seems to have long-term efficacy. It may, however, cause an unwanted drowsiness during waking hours.

A variety of other problems may be aggravated by hypnotics:

1 The failure of some controls in the cortex may lead to early confusion with excitement, anxiety, restlessness, and stimulation. Cerebral anoxia may result from impaired respiratory function or low output cardiac failure and lowered blood pressure, thus confusing drug action with pathological processes that require specific treatment. Sedatives depressing cardiac and respiratory functions should be used carefully, if at all, in patients with arteriosclerotic cerebral vessels.

2 Slow accumulation of drug in brain tissue, attributable to slowed metabolism and excretion, may lead to apathy, torpor, and possibly a reversed day-night rhythm. Dosage and timing are important, especially in old people with deterioration of brain function. Bedtime barbiturates may continue to act through the following day by causing drowsiness, but as night approaches the patient may again become restless and confused. It is best to start with small doses given early in the evening.

3 Insomnia may be due to a full bladder or rectum. Sedatives may aggravate the retention and worsen the insomnia.

4 Oversedation resulting in immobility may predispose the patient to osteoporosis, contractures, and pressure sores in a very short time.

5 Even moderate doses of barbiturates may intensify the rigidity of parkinsonism.

MAJOR TRANQUILIZERS

Phenothiazines stimulate or depress normal physiologic actions of nerve cells in the various parts of the central nervous system, the total effect on an old person consisting of the sum of stimulation and inhibition in a brain in partial decline. The following considerations are of particular concern in the elderly:

1 They are particularly susceptible to cholinergic blockade, which may aggravate constipation. In addition, many old people taking phenothiazines will have an unpleasant dryness of the mouth that may cause trouble with teeth, gums, or dentures.

2 Extrapyramidal symptoms occur in about 50 percent of elderly people who use this group of drugs. Such symptoms consist of uncontrollable involuntary movements, sometimes grotesque. These movements are under the control of brain centers apart from the "pyramidal" centers. These brain centers control purposeful coordinated movements such as writing or chewing. The type of extrapyramidal effect which occurs is age-related. Younger patients have a

greater likelihood of dyskinesia, which is difficulty in performing voluntary movements; middle-aged persons tend toward akathisia, an uncontrolled restlessness which is a precursor to parkinsonism; older persons tend toward parkinsonism with its muscle rigidity, weakness, and coarse tremors. However, age is less important than the chemical structure and the size of the dose in accounting for unpleasant drug reactions. The piperazines cause a relatively high frequency of extrapyramidal symptoms. Fortunately, most ambulatory geriatric patients do not require doses capable of inducing neurologic symptoms. Once symptoms develop, however, they tend to be permanent, requiring administration of antiparkinsonism drugs long after the phenothiazine has been discontinued.

Tardive dyskinesia is an involuntary, persistent, rhythmical, purposeless movement of lips, tongue, and jaw. It may or may not be accompanied by smacking, drooling, and grimacing, When severe, it may interfere with talking or swallowing. To people who are overly fastidious or naive, tardive dyskinesia can be repulsive. So far as is known, tardive dyskinesia and other extrapyramidal disorders are due to alterations of certain neurotransmitters in brain centers. Extrapyramidal movements sometimes can be controlled by reducing the dose of the offending drug, by changing drugs, by giving drugs that are useful in Parkinson's disease (to be discussed later), or by stopping the phenothiazine altogether. Sometimes, however, especially in tardive dyskinesia, the abnormal movements will be aggravated by drug withdrawal.

Why, then, are phenothiazines used at all? Simply, their benefits outweigh their disadvantages. They, more than any other advance in psychiatry, have enabled many highly disturbed people to lead relatively normal lives. It is when such patients get old that the undesirable effects are apt to show up. Then, too, people who have never used drugs also get extrapyramidal symptoms. A British study showed that one-fourth of all patients with tardive dyskinesia were never exposed to phenothiazines. It can develop from hypoxia due to poisoning or to severe respiratory embarrassment.

Orthostatic hypotension, a potentially dangerous fall in blood pressure when a person stands, may occur in old people taking phenothiazines. Again, the condition does ōccasionally occur without medication in feeble old people, but the chance that a faint or a fall will occur is greater with phenothiazine medication. Hip fractures are common from falls during these dizzy spells. Hypotension occurs even more often with the piperidyl and dimethylaminopropyl derivatives. Both the dimethylaminopropyl phenothiazines and the thioxanthenes are potent alpha-adrenergic antagonists as compared with the weaker piperazines and butyrophenones. The hypotension can also lead to myocardial infarction. Patients should be monitored closely, especially when medication is started. Supine and standing blood-pressure measurements should be made before and after a test dose in older patients.

As with any tranquilizing drug, overtranquilization may lead to stagnation of blood in legs and feet, phlebitis, and thrombosis. Prolonged therapy with drugs with autonomic effects leading to xerostomia (dry mouth) can cause parotid infection. Patients unable to tend to themselves should be kept well-hydrated and be given good oral care.

Chlorpromazine, the first widely used phenothiazine and still among the most useful, is especially apt to cause jaundice that may be indistinguishable from more serious liver diseases.

In our experience the most useful phenothiazine drug is thioridazine (Mellaril). It relieves the agitation that nearly always accompanies depression in the elderly. If a patient is hostile or frightened in new surroundings he or she may be quieted and be made amenable to reassurance and support following the use of Mellaril. In old people with serious heart or lung disease, agitation and restlessness can be dangerous. In such a situation, sedation with a drug such as Mellaril may be lifesaving. The drug should be given in a dose large enough to quiet the patient. Then the dose can be adjusted downward to allow the patient to function at his highest level.

Haldol, a butyrophenone, is advertised as useful to quiet unruly patients. In our experience there are better drugs for this purpose, ones which are more predictable and less expensive. For old people who have hallucinations, however, Haldol frequently will relieve this most disturbing of psychiatric symptoms without making the patient drowsy.

ANTIDEPRESSANTS

Before discussing antidepressant drugs, we should talk briefly about depression in the elderly. We don't mean temporary gloom such as people may have from time to time on a cold, rainy day. We mean a persistent pathological disorder marked by despondency that may lead to suicide. Most often the symptoms—hopelessness, sleeplessness, withdrawal, changed eating habits, and loss of a sense of proportion—are far out of proportion to actual circumstances. A frequent cause or effect is diminished sexual drive, but here, as in many psychiatric illnesses, causes and effects are hard to sort out. In some patients the only evidence of depression is that they become crotchety and overly sensitive. Most depressions get better in a few weeks without treatment.

When a depressed patient finally goes to the doctor and complains of irritability and poor sleeping, the symptoms may be taken too lightly. If the physician is hurried or does not understand the underlying depression, he or she may prescribe a minor tranquilizer such as Valium. If the depression is not self-limiting, as many are, the medicine is apt to aggravate the symptoms, to cause confusion, and to lead to a faulty diagnosis of senile dementia. In a busy geriatrics practice, overmedication for mild nervousness often leads to protracted illness. Then, a patient may be referred to a psychiatrist who may not understand that the chief problem is not a relatively minor depression but medication. Finally, the patient may be referred to a physician who understands depression in old people, stops the medicine entirely, and allows the patient to improve. Such events don't occur every day in the life of a geriatrician, but they do occur about every month. Assuming the physicians are perceptive, that they make accurate diagnoses, that they give assurance and moral support, what then? Patients may improve simply with reassurance and support. More likely, antidepressant medications will be prescribed.

The tricyclic antidepressants—so-called because of their chemical structure—are used most often. These are very useful drugs, but we believe they are used promiscuously. By this we mean that they are prescribed without enough human considerations. When used in conjunction with acceptance, understanding, and moral support they can be helpful. Indeed, if human qualities are generously shared, antidepressants often become unnecessary.

The dibenzocycloheptenes, especially, amitriptyline (Elavil), should be used cautiously in cardiovascular disease because of induced hypotension and electrocardiographic changes. Other cardiotoxic effects incluce tachycardia and extrasystoles. They may cause transient insommia, and amitriptyline may cause a potentially dangerous unsteadiness of gait.

Doxepin does not produce changes in the electrocardiagram and has the fewest anticholinergic effects of any tricyclic antidepressant, traits especially desired in patients with lowered gastric motility, constipation, or a high risk of glaucoma.

Monoamine oxidase (MAO) inhibitors are not used as much as formerly because of their interaction with certain foods and other drugs (see Chapter 5). We can think of no good reason for their use in old people.

SUMMARY

So far in this chapter we have written of functional conditions of mind or mood, that is, those conditions which are not necessarily reflected in structural alteration or disease in the central nervous system. In doing so we are aware that in elderly people the precise definition of what is functional and what is organic is often difficult or impossible. The two possibilities coexist to the point that only the most experienced and perceptive person may be able to sort out possible causes for aberrant behavior. In our experience, only psychiatrists who have taken a special interest in old people can be of much help.

Let us return to Mrs. O. (Chapter 3), whose problem was not organic brain disease or depression. It was logical to suppose that her loss of appetite was due to depression, but this was definitely wrong. It was logical that she could have had a chronic brain syndrome, but she didn't. On the other hand, people who forget their own name, who do not recognize their own spouse, who become untidy, and who lose control of bladder and bowels surely have something "organic" going on in the central nervous system. They are at opposite ends of a bipolar scheme:

$$\text{Functional} \longleftrightarrow \text{Organic}$$

Added to either pole may be stresses or other influences such as loneliness, grief, fear, impaired health, reduced social status, poor nutrition, alcohol, one or more drugs, etc. The problem of sorting out what is treatable and what is not is formidable.

Since the aging brain is a source of such misery and misunderstanding, we believe it deserves further discussion and have devoted the following chapter to it.

Chapter 9

Organic Brain Syndromes

The aging brain is often afflicted by social, psychological, and physiological problems. These arise from the aging process, the stresses of life, diseases throughout the body, drugs, and even nutritional deficiencies.

An *organic* brain syndrome, then, involves a measurable loss of intelligence through impaired brain function or neuronal loss. And the older the person the more likely it is that there will be some brain damage resulting in lesser intellect, orientation, and judgment. We frequently see people with poor memories who cannot remember the day of the week, do not always know where they are, and may appear on the wrong day for an appointment. Impaired brain function is a hallmark of senility whether it occurs at age 50 or 100.

The syndrome sometimes involves psychosis. The psychosis may arise from dementia or from such brain-damaging factors as alcohol, infection, or nutritional deficiencies. Severe dementia may resemble schizophrenia or depression. Careful questioning can differentiate between true depression and a genuine loss of intellect and orientation.[1] The people may become psychotic and require physical restraint to prevent them from injuring themselves or others.

At this point we should define a few terms.

Delirium Delirium is an acute, frequently reversible, frequently alarming, and potentially dangerous mental derangement which is particularly apt to occur in older people. It is manifested by delusions, hallucinations, tremors, hyperactivity, agitation, disorientation, hostility, fright, sweating, flushing, fever, or some combination thereof. Delirium is subject to many complications in the elderly because it may add to the burden of the already overburdened cardiovascular system. Delirium is caused either by the failure of the metabolic support of the brain or by drugs or toxins that depress cerebral metabolism. Delirium is not so much a syndrome as it is the effect on the brain by some substance. By resolving the underlying problem, the delirum may be resolved.

Dementia Dementia is the degeneration of higher cortical neurons, resulting in loss of intellect. This loss of neurons, usually in the parietal, temporal, and frontal lobes of the cerebral cortex, is chronic, irreversible, and progressive. Dementia is one of the most common syndromes afflicting the elderly. Each year about 2.3 percent of those over 65 years of age have to be institutionalized and about 60,000 to 90,000 die with dementia. This does not include those over 65 years of age whose death certificate may list only the immediate cause of death.[2,3] Some claim that dementia markedly reduces life span, but because it usually occurs in the later stages of senescence, the person with dementia does tend to have a relatively short survival. Upon looking at the remaining life span of those with and without dementia, there may not be much difference. Also, because dementia is often considered untreatable, the lack of treatment may contribute to the high mortality.[4]

Acute versus Chronic These terms refer to the potential for reversability. When the condition is irreversible because brain cells are dead, it is *chronic*. When the condition is reversible, it is *acute*. Complicating the evaluation of a patient may be the coexistence of the two. The chronic brain syndrome of senile dementia may be worsened by an acute episode involving too many barbiturates or some metabolic disorder.[5]

DIAGNOSIS

The first step in treating an organic brain syndrome is to diagnose the illness properly. The interplay of functional and organic must be determined and differentiated. Since some of these syndromes are treatable, they must be properly diagnosed. Many symptoms and complications can be relieved if recognized.

One diagnostic aid is the electroencephalogram (EEG), and several changes here correlate well with cerebral disturbances. Mild slowing and disorganization of the waking background in the EEG may indicate mild encephalopathy and decreased intellectural functioning. This occurs with cerebrovascular disease and cerebral atrophy, in which cortical metabolism is inadequate. This pattern may also indicate such metabolic disorders as hypoxia, hypoglycemia, hypothyroidism, and hepatic or renal disease as well as drug toxicity. A predominantly low-voltage, fast rhythm may be seen along with the confusion of torpor seen in toxicity from barbiturates and related drugs. A diffuse moderate to high-voltage, fast activity may occur with toxicity from amphetamines.

In the elderly person, the dominant alpha rhythm is slower and has diminished amplitude. The general EEG changes in senility include background slowing, a less-responsive graph, and synchronous slow waves. So the strongest association with senility is a slowing EEG pattern.

A depressed person, who may appear demented, has either a normal EEG or, possibly, much low-voltage beta activity instead of diffuse slowing.[6,7]

In recent years, computerized axial tomography, a highly technical x-ray procedure, has helped to diagnose and guide treatment in mental disease in old people.

By no means do we feel that every old, demented person should be subjected to these costly procedures, which in our opinion are helpful only to the occasional patient. The procedures should be used not to satisfy curiosity but only to guide treatment in borderline cases.

THE CAUSES OF DELIRIUM

I Toxic psychoses
   A Toxic psychoses associated with the drugs or poisons.
      1 *Barbiturates.* These can make a person dull, sluggish, sleepy, slow in speech, and disturbed in thought and judgment. The attention span narrows, and the person is easily upset and becomes petulant, quarrelsome, irritable, morose, hostile, and even paranoid.
      2 *Amphetamines.* Amphetamines can cause a disorder that mimics schizophrenia.
      3 *Antidiabetics.* Hypoglycemic effects in the brain can appear when the elderly diabetic's blood sugar is lowered into the "normal" range of 100 to 150 milligrams per 100 milliliters. These patients tolerate blood glucose levels of 150 to 250 milligrams per 100 milliliters much better than they do the lower range, where irreversible brain damage may occur.[8] Chlorpropamide may cause inappropriate antidiuretic hormone secretion, leading to water intoxication.
      4 *Diuretics.* Their use can lead to dehydration, electrolyte imbalance, and confusion. Severe hypokalemia may be accompanied by anorexia, gastrointestinal discomfort, and muscle weakness so great that walking is difficult. Impaired mental function occurs in many cases when serum potassium is less than 3.5 milliequivalents per liter.
      5 *Hypotensives.* The hypertensive's brain seems to reset its autoregulatory mechanism controlling the relationship between

cerebral blood pressure and cerebral blood flow. There is a higher setting. So antihypertensive drugs which produce a normal blood pressure may cause either general or focal hypoperfusion.[10] After the age of 70, only malignant hypertension or hypertensive heart failure should be treated. Both of these are uncommon.

6 *Antiparkinsonism drugs*. Changes in neurotransmitter chemistry in the cerebral hemispheres comparable to those in the corpus striatum may produce acute confusion within hours.

   a *Anticholinergic-type*. Patients entering their sixties and seventies who were once able to tolerate large doses of these drugs may suddenly become increasingly sensitive to anticholinergics. Early signs of intolerance include mild confusion, nightmares, and increased absentmindedness. This may progress to more severe mental confusion, visual and aural hallucinations, and, possibly, paranoid delusions.

   b *Levodopa* is also less well tolerated in the elderly. Mental symptoms may include elation, depression, markedly damaged cognitive perceptions, disorientation, paranoid fixations, and agitation. Fortunately these problems are not universal. These people seem to tolerate only about 80% of the dose for a younger person.[11−13]

7 *Digoxin*. Digoxin−induced confusion is probably due to a direct action on the central nervous system. Additionally, digoxin−induced cardiac arrhythmias may present as brain failure. There may be depression, anorexia, irritability, weakness, and drowsiness.[14]

8 *Phenothiazines*. Of 236 patients admitted to one psychogeriatric service, 15% had mental disorders directly attributable to psychotropic drugs. Confusion is especially likely if the phenothiazine is administered with anticholinergic-type antiparkinsonism such as trihexyphenidyl (Artane, Tremin), tricyclic antidepressants (Endep, Elavil, Tofranil, Aventyl), and, possibly, some antihistamines.[15]

9 *Benzodiazepines*. Relatively small doses of diazepam (Valium) cause stuporous sleep, sluggishness, drowsiness, and impaired walking in geriatric patients. Valium can also cause a small but significant degree of depression, decreased memory and intellectual function, and fatigue in men over 75 years.[16,17] Flurazepam (Dalmane) has been implicated in inducing a high incidence of ataxia, confusion, and hallucinations in institutionalized geriatric patients.[18] Because of the long half-life of active flurazepam metabolites (50 to 100 hours) and a significant drug level for five to six times this, problems may not appear for as long as three weeks after beginning the drug.[19] The onset of symptoms is gradual. Let us reiterate several basic concepts concerning *all* hypnotics: The underlying cause of insomnia should be treated, low doses should be administered only intermittently and for short

periods of time, and they should be used only if other drug and nondrug therapy is not successful.[18]

10   *Narcotics.* Narcotics easily cause mental confusion and worsen any other mental deficiencies.[20] It is appalling that many old people in hospitals are rendered delirious from the ill-advised use of such drugs as morphine, and meperidine (Demerol). Often the standard preanesthetic medications are ordered for old people who are then given an anesthetic for an operation. It is no wonder that many old people become deranged postoperatively.

11   *Alcohol.* Delirium tremens or alcoholic delirium is not infrequent in elderly drinkers. We have been surprised on occasion at the onset of delirium in otherwise minor illnesses. Only then does it become known that the patient was a chronic drinker of alcohol, though "alcoholism" would not be acknowledged. After all, the patient had never been drunk in his or her life.

12   *Indomethacin, steroids, anticholinergics, reserpine, and phenytoin.* These drugs cause various symptoms ranging from depression to psychosis.

B   *Metabolic imbalances*

1   *Hypercalcemia.* This can cause lethargy and confusion. Hypercalcemia may be secondary to cancers of the lung, breast, and other tissues; multiple myelomas; thiazides; Paget's disease; immobilization; primary hyperparathyroidism; and, possibly, great excesses of calcium-containing antacids.[21]

2   *Hyperglycemia.* Hyperglycemia can occur in diabetic ketoacidosis, lactic acidosis, and nonacidotic hyperosmolar syndrome.

3   *Hypoglycemia.* Hypoglycemia may be caused by insulin or antidiabetic drugs. It may not be accompanied by increased sympathetic activity such as tachycardia, panting, and sweating. The speech slurs, the behavior is bizarre, and the person becomes confused and sleepy.

4   *Hypothyroidism*

5   *Hyperthyroidism.* In the elderly patient this may appear as apathy or depression, i.e., "apathetic hyperthyroidism." There may also be a large weight loss and cardiovascular disease.

6   *Hypernatremia* (hyperosmolar). This may be secondary to poor fluid intake, excessive sweating, concussion, or the use of hypertonic sodium chloride or high-protein tube feeding.

7   *Hyponatremia.* Hyponatremia may arise from disorders of antidiuretic hormone secretion such as in bronchogenic carcinoma, cerebrovascular accidents, and wounds. Water shifts into cells, which become overhydrated. The function of the cells is impaired, and mental processes are clouded.

8   *Azotemia.* This may arise from renal disease or acute bladder overload. The latter may come from the use of such diuretics as furosemide and ethacrynic acid.

II Nutrition. Over 10% of the elderly have simultaneous deficiencies of at least four vitamins: thiamine, riboflavin, ascorbic acid, and folic acid. These and other deficiencies may be involved in central nervous system dysfunction. As we shall see when looking at the various therapies used or reported for the organic brain syndromes, vitamins have relieved symptoms in a few patients.

III Tumors. Tumors may impair mental function by causing increased intracranial pressure or by causing metabolic imbalances.

IV Hepatic factors. Factors such as hepatitis and cirrhosis may cause mental impairment since there may be inadequate excretion of metabolic wastes. This is particularly apt to occur in old people who have livers damaged by alcohol.

V Cardiac factors. Mental impairment results from decreased output of blood. Among the elderly, 13% of those having a myocardial infarction have confusion as a major brain symptom. Brain failure may be one of the first signs of heart disease, especially when there are disturbances of cardiac rhythm.

VI Febrile conditions. Any fever, especially one due to infections of the central nervous system such as meningitis, may produce delirium.

VII Decreased pulmonary function. Due to chronic lung disease with hypoxia or hypercapnea, it may cause impaired mental function.

VIII Low-pressure hydrocephalus. This is a syndrome of rapidly appearing dementia, ataxia, and incontinence. Brain operations appear to have helped a few patients in their early seventies, but the operation has not found wide acceptance.

IX Depression. We discussed depression and its treatment in an earlier chapter. We include it in this classification because it is frequently abrupt in onset, treatable, and is not due to organic brain damage, although it many be concurrent. Sometimes depressions are called nervous breakdowns or rundown conditions. They often lead to operations of questionable value since they can masquerade as other ailments. People with depressions may receive perverse satisfaction in avoiding the issue of depression by ill-advised treatment. Unfortunately, many physicians are not as aware as they should be of the symptoms of depression. About 5% of people over 65 years of age have a well-defined depressive illness, according to most surveys. If, however, one looks carefully for symptoms of depression, such as fatigue, anxiety, poor sleeping, and low spirits, depression can be diagnosed in about 11% of old people at some time.[22]

Depression may often arise from the various losses suffered by the elderly. Old people are subject to many illnesses with chronic physical and psychological disabilities, sensory losses, and general decline. They are often socially and economically deprived. And they are often lonely.

Various biological factors can contribute to depression in the elderly. Increasing levels of monoamine oxidase in plasma, hindbrain, and platelets cause lower levels of norepinephrine and dopamine. (MAO is inversely proportional to estrogen; at menopause, estrogen declines and MAO increases.) A declining thyroid function and decreased pituitary responsiveness to thyroid-releasing factor (from the hypothalamus) also make it more difficult to cope with stress. Deprivation of REM sleep may cause depression, and older people with their changing sleep patterns spend less time in REM sleep.[23,24]

Neurotic or reactive depressions are chronic and not usually self-limiting. The person is apathetic and withdrawn, feels empty and exhausted, and is difficult to engage in activities. These people regress and become demanding. This state is often mistaken for senile dementia.[25,26]

Some old character traits may predispose people to depression. For instance, obsessive persons with controlled hostility are more prone to depression.[27]

All these deliriums are generally relieved by treating the underlying cause, whether by reducing drug dosages, improving the diet, or treating the disease.

THE CAUSES OF DEMENTIA

We now turn from the types of delirium to the dementias, organic psychoses, chronic organic brain syndromes, call them what you will. There has been a confusion of terms which has led to a confusion in understanding of just what happens to the aging brain. Senility has taken on a pejorative connotation that causes old people to lose self-esteem. If an adolescent is forgetful or unthought-ful, the tendency is to blame it on the youth without rejecting the child. In old people, simple forgetfulness may unjustly become a signal for drastic change in their lives. Notwithstanding this demurrer, however, the fact is there is a loss of brain substance with aging. The question then becomes: What is disease and what is simply a process of aging? The answers are still confused and we will probably not discuss them here. We merely wish to point out that one should be very cautious in categorizing an old person whose intellectual functioning may be impaired. We have often seen old people regain a high level of function after their general health and sense of place are improved.

At one time senile dementia was believed to be caused by reduced blood flow to the brain, and so senile dementia was synonymous with cerebral ar-teriosclerosis. Most normal elderly people do have altered cerebral vasculature but a relatively good cerebral autoregulation. Some with irreversible arteri-osclerosis and severe anomalies have good gray-matter flow and vasomotor reactivity. In any event, there does not seem to be a good correlation between the loss of mental abilities and cerebral circulatory and metabolic defects.[28,29]

Still, many older persons with no apparent mental decline or with only mild symptoms may have arteriosclerosis or some other circulatory insufficiency caus-ing cerebral hypoxia. This hypoxia can eventually damage cerebral tissue and reduce cerebral metabolism. So when the organic brain syndrome is quite appar-ent, the demand has been reduced to meet the supply. The damage is now irreversible; improvement cannot occur.

It is now recognized that there is another source of senile dementia, which involves a primary degeneration of the brain cells rather than a declining blood flow to the brain. This disease, *Alzheimer's disease*, is reflected in about a 23 percent decline in average cerebral blood flow and cerebral oxidative metabolism, chiefly in the gray matter. This reduced flow is related to the degree of mental impairment, but the reactivity of the vessels is normal. The neuronal degeneration and reduced brain function result in less cerebral metabolism which in turn results in less blood flow to the area. This decline in regional cerebral blood flow is the result of brain cell destruction and not the other way around.[30,31]

How does this work? Brain metabolism produces carbon dioxide. This carbon dioxide in the blood produces carbonic acid, which lowers the pH of extracellular fluid, causing relaxation of the smooth muscles of the arterioles. Increasing blood flow washes out carbon dioxide faster and raises the pH of the extracellular fluid, and this causes vasoconstriction. This autoregulation of cerebrovascular resistance maintains a constant flow despite variations in perfusion pressure. Above a critical perfusion pressure of about 60 mmHg, blood flow to the brain is pretty much regulated by carbon dioxide produced by nervous system metabolism. Thus when there is little metabolism producing carbon dioxide, there is little blood flow to the area.

A reduced cerebral oxygen supply, as with strokes, upsets this regulatory mechanism by causing lactic acidosis. Acidosis in turn produces prolonged vasodilation and increased blood flow to the area. So blood flow to such an area becomes a direct function of perfusion pressure.

There are many sympathetic and parasympathetic nerves in the larger cerebral vessels, but they do not seem to cause more than a 10 to 15 percent change in cerebral blood flow. Sympathetic fibers generally end before they reach the intracerebral vasculature.[32]

We can now be more specific about the circulatory subtypes and Alzheimer's disease. We shall discuss their differentiation and their statistics.

I Circulatory subtypes
  A *Cerebral arteriosclerosis.* Arterial changes occur in about one-third of patients with organic brain syndrome and contribute to the pathology in another 10%. Diffuse damage causes a reduced level of awareness or reduced mental activity. Specific, or focal, damage to parts of the brain causes characteristic disturbances in such actions as swallowing, in vision, or in strength in specific areas such as the arms, legs, or face. There may be sudden confusion, incoherence, weakness, restlessness, hallucinations, and delirium, followed by a gradual decline in mental capacity. These patients do not have the profound mental decay seen in those with Alzheimer's disease.
  B *Extracranial arterial occlusive disease.* This disease may also develop, producing cerebral vascular insufficiency, which may cause visual disturbances, vertigo, and sensory and motor defects. A not infrequent example of this kind of disturbance occurs in the carotid arteries, which occasionally may be amenable to surgical treatment.

    C *Multi–infarct dementias* are caused by numerous small infarctions with a step-by-step deterioration, leading to a condition resembling Alzheimer's disease.

    D Finally there are a variety of other circulatory disturbances such as cerebral emboli, cardiac decompensation, hypertensive encephalopathy, pulmonary emboli, cardiac dysrhythmias, and subdural hematomas. All these conditions may possibly be corrected or improved by treatment.

II Alzheimer's disease. This is a primary cellular degeneration. Microscopically there is a great loss of neurons, there are neurofibrillatory tangles represented by two neurofilaments wrapped together, and there are granulovacuolar changes representing degeneration of the remaining neurons. Between the cells are "senile plaques" composed of enlarged abnormal nerve fibers and synaptic endings with degenerated mitochondria and containing an amyloid core.[3] There are at least four proposed causes of Alzheimer's Disease.

    A There may be a genetic factor. More of a certain gene is found in these patients than in the remainder of the population.

    B Slow-acting viruses analogous to those causing scrapie, kuru, and Creutzfeldt-Jakob disease may be involved.

    C Because amyloid, the primary constituent of the senile plaques, is probably derived from immunoglobulines, immunologic mechanisms have been postulated.

    D Aluminum may act as a cytotoxic factor. Aluminum is toxic to neurons and can cause neurofibrillatory tangles similar but not identical to those found in Alzheimer brains. These afflicted brains also have more aluminum than brains without the disease. Whether the aluminum causes the tangles or whether some other factor in the degenerating brain collects the aluminum is unknown.[33]

Certain enzymatic and neurotransmitter changes have also been observed in the demented brain. In both aging and degenerative brain diseases, certain nerve cells, especially cholinergic ones, are most affected. There is some question about whether degeneration of presynaptic nerve terminals is involved and whether a deficiency of acetylcholine is characteristic of the disease. Acetylcholinesterase activity declines. Levodopa decarboxylase and glutamic acid decarboxylase (GAD) activity decline. These enzymes are involved in the formation of the neurotransmitters dopamine, norepinephrine, and γ-aminobutyric acid (GABA). Thus the activity of these transmitters and inhibitory neurotransmitters tend to be reduced. On the other hand, there are increasing amounts of acid phosphatase, lactic dehydrogenase, malate dehydrogenase, and cytochrome oxidase.[35]

As with the cerebrovascular changes in mentally healthy persons, the senile degenerative changes of plaques, tangles, and cerebral softening can also be found in the brains of mentally active older persons.

To gain some idea of the extent to which cerebrovascular changes and primary cellular degeneration contribute to the overall incidence of senile dementia, let us look at a study of autopsy results. Alzheimer's disease accounted for 50 percent of the dementias and was a considerable factor in an additional 24 percent. Massive ischemic lesions *alone* accounted for 12 percent of the dementias, and an additional 8 percent also had massive ischemic lesions. Sixteen percent had considerable ischemic lesions. About 4 percent had no lesions but suffered a diffuse cell death.[36]

Arteriosclerotic dementia is the more frequent ante-mortem diagnosis because small strokes and hypertension are events brought to the attention of the physician. On the other hand, the number of brain cells declines from youth onward but not at a rate such as to interfere with cerebral functioning and raise the question of dementia. From the above figures it appears that in only 4 percent of autopsies on patients with dementia is general diffuse cell death severe enough to be responsible for the dementia. Rather, in middle and especially old age, when the brain cell population has been greatly reduced, diffuse cell death, cerebrovascular changes, and other senile processes may combine. The total effect depends on the type of pathologic process, its location in the brain, and its extent.

Differentiation of Cellular Degeneration and Vascular Disease

There are two general methods of differentiating the dementias of cellular degeneration from vascular disease, a process that is often difficult and fraught with error.

Clinical Aspects *Vascular disease* usually occurs in men in their late sixties. There is a patchy dementia with gross mental deterioration but in which insight and personality are often preserved. Most likely the person will be hypertensive. Certainly, dementia is unusual under the age of 60 without severe hypertension. The disease progresses by stages or episodes over about 5 years. Death is frequently from ischemic heart disease.[37]

In *Alzheimer's disease,* primary tissue degeneration, as far as we can tell, is more common in women and may be inherited. The condition may begin at any time from the thirties to extreme old age. Blood pressure is normal. Brain, muscle, and viscera waste away.

Even without cerebrovascular impairment there can be extensive intellectual impairment from heart disease, hypertension, reduced pulmonary function, and peripheral arteriosclerosis.[38]

Cerebral Blood Flow and Metabolism Although old age alone is not absolutely equated with a declining cerebral blood flow and metabolism, decline from degenerative disease is so widespread that it seems that way.

As blood flows through the brain, the brain extracts a certain quantity of oxygen and glucose so that there is a noticeable difference of these between the arterial and venous blood. This is more simply referred to as the A V difference.

If blood flow declines in a healthy brain, perhaps because of some vascular defect such as infarction or atherosclerosis, the brain extracts a greater percentage of glucose and oxygen from the lesser blood supply. Consequently the A V difference increases and cerebral metabolism remains normal.

If the blood flow declines to 15 to 18 milliliters per 100 grams of tissue per minute, the cells remain alive but become anoxic and nonfunctional. Below 10 milliliters per 100 grams per minute, the cells die. So initially an improved flow of blood improves the performance of these cells and the person's performance. But after a point, the cells die and cannot return to life.

In early primary cellular degeneration, as in Alzheimer's disease, the A V difference remains the same or may *decrease*, and cerebral blood flow slowly declines as a response to less metabolic activity in the brain.[39]

So in the early stages of dementia, blood-flow studies and measurements of A V differences in glucose and oxygen can differentiate the two basic types of mental deterioration.

THE CLINICAL COURSE OF DEMENTIA

The onset of dementia is insidious. There may be mental depression ranging from inconsequential to marked. More noticeable, aside from this depression, is the disturbed memory or a failure of perception. Recent occurrences may be forgotten although recall of the more distant past may be fairly well preserved. Routine tasks and functions are forgotten. Interests become more self-centered, and people become emotionally unstable and have difficulty in understanding, responding to, and remembering new experiences. Some may become agitated, paranoid, and have dreadful hallucinations.

As the disease progresses, intellectual functions decline. The ability to comprehend and think can be reduced. Although routine activities can be performed, new procedures or even slight revisions of old task become difficult or impossible. People lose interest in more and more things.

Although about one-half of patients with dementia seem depressed, others have a euphoria or an unjustified feeling of joy. They feel quite confident and are not aware of their derangement. They cannot understand why others are so concerned. (Another proof of a corollary of Murphy's law: When all seems to be going well, you have overlooked something.)

Personality changes can be quite varied. These may be exaggerations of the person's former personality. The slightly obsessional person may become more obsessional and fussy. Conversely, the quiet person may become uninhibited, loud, and aggressive. We have seen a saintly Sunday school teacher become the dirtiest talker one could imagine. As the degeneration continues, patients may lose the ability to express themselves, to recognize common objects, or do anything useful. By the end, which may be as long as ten years after the onset of dementia, there is a total breakdown in intellect and personality, and the person is totally dependent on others. He or she must be fed, dressed, and cleaned by others. Bowel and bladder control is gone. These people are little more than breathing vegetables or old infants in their behavior.

In addition to these two major types of dementia, another type should be mentioned. A history of alcoholism is frequent among demented persons. Patients with alcoholic dementia have many of the symptoms we have described above. Many patients in institutions and veteran's facilities, and old alcoholics who function on the fringe of society, have organic brain disease caused by alcohol ingestion over a period of years. Once alcoholic brain disease is established, it rarely improves after alcohol is witheld.

There are two syndromes supposedly characteristic of chronic alcoholic brain disease: (1) Korsakoff's syndrome, manifested by confabulation, and (2) Wernicke's syndrome, manifested chiefly by incoordination. Often, these syndromes will become apparent in the forties and fifties and if they do, alcoholism should be suspected. Recently, it has been shown that Korsakoff's syndrome is due to a genetic defect in which an enzyme necessary for the metabolism of thiamine becomes deficient in alcoholics. This discovery may be a clue to the cause of other cases of organic brain syndrome.

So, as we can see, dementia in the elderly is due to Alzheimer changes, to impaired circulation, to alcohol, or to a combination of these. Brain cells may be unaffected, mildly to severely impaired, or dead. It is likely that varying mixtures of these can account for the varying results of drug efficacy in different studies. Again, it is really difficult to categorize the organic brain syndromes, especially in individual patients. The difficulty is overcome by combining them under the term *chronic organic brain syndromes*.

TREATMENT OF DEMENTIA

There has been a tendency to assume that the chronic dementias are untreatable. Such a fatalistic attitude, of course, does not do justice to many attractive, loving old people whose minds are gone. Many old people with dementia are like winsome children, amiable and cooperative. They have often reminded us of one of the beatitudes: "Blessed are the pure of heart." The problem is in finding drugs and procedures that are safe and effective. Unfortunately, very few are both.

There is much conflicting evidence conerning the values of vasodilators, hydrogenated ergot alkaloids, anticoagulants, hyperbaric oxygen, and a few others. This section will present the rationale for each of these and some of the results.

Medical Letter gives an evaluation of all such drugs. It says "...progressive degenerative changes in the brain itself and not faulty circulation through atherosclerotic blood vessels is the cause of mental deterioration or dementia in the elderly. Nothing works very well and improving mental and behavioral symptoms is best done by improving social and occupation circumstances."[40] This may or may not be so.

The methods of treating the dementias may be categorized as follows.

I Drug therapy
    A Improved brain function
       1 Yeast ribonucleic acid (RNA)
       2 Neurotransmitters
       3 Hydrogenated ergot alkaloids
    B Increased oxygen to the brain
       1 Hyperbaric oxygen
       2 Vasodilators
       3 Anticoagulants
       4 Carbonic anhydrase inhibitors
    C Symptom suppression
       1 Antipsychotics
       2 Antianxiety drugs
       3 Sedative-hypnotics
       4 Antidepressants
    D Miscellaneous
II Nondrug therapy
    A Reality orientation
    B Behavior modification
    C Ergonomics
    D Normalization

Drug Therapy

Improved Brain Function

Yeast Ribonucleic Acid (RNA)   Some improvement has been reported in some patients, especially among those with arteriosclerotic–induced memory changes. There is little or no improvement in the presenile and senile, and nothing has really been proven. It is possible the benefit could have come from the extra attention given the patients.[41–43]

Neurotransmitters   Senile dementia is often associated with the latter stages of Parkinson's disease, and it has been observed that many of these demented Parkinson's patients are either mentally improved or worsened after treatment with levodopa.[44,45] The failure of levodopa often can be ascribed to the advanced state of the disease, so that the exogenously administered neurotransmitter precursor cannot be converted to the neurotransmitter, or the neurons cannot transmit from one brain area to the next.[46,47] Thus, a favorable response is related to the person's residual resources when therapy begins. And conversely, in some, levodopa may worsen the symptoms by reducing intellectual functions even further and may cause paranoid or agitated behavior.[48]

Tyrosine and tryptophan are amino acids and precursors to such neurotransmitters as dopamine, norepinephrine, epinephrine, and 1,5-hydroxytryptamine. A combination of these precursors were fed to demented patients with the idea that the production of the neurotransmitters might be enhanced. There was no improvement in those with Alzheimer's disease and only slight improvement in one of three multi-infarct dementia patients.

It is also interesting to note that none of the patients deteriorated during this study. Better results may have been obtained by using urinary excretion data to pinpoint the precise neurotransmitter deficit. Also, unfortunately for this study, tryptophan, not 1,5-hydroxytryptamine was used in this study, the 1,5-hydroxtyryptamine (serotonin) precursor of choice.[15] Although 1,5-hydroxytryptophan does increase brain serotonin, there is not an appreciable increase in the levels in the serotoninergic neurons in the brain-stem raphe nucleus, and the regional brain distribution of serotonin and its metabolite 5-hydroxyindoleacetic acid (5-HIAA) are abnormal after 5-hydroxytryptophan is given. This indicates it does not act in a physiological manner, and so exogenously administered 5-hydroxytryptophan may not be a natural precursor to serotonin.[49,50]

This kind of experiment is an example of approaches that do no harm and may do a great deal of good for hundreds of thousands of people.

Dihydrogenated Ergot Alkaloids (DHEA) (Hydergine, Circanol, Deapril-ST)   DHEA, a combination of ergot alkaloids, was originally believed to act as a cerebral vasodilator. It does have such an effect, but its action is primarily on ganglion cell metabolism. There are several observations of interest here.

As cerebral blood flow and oxygen supply decline, the cell shifts from aerobic pyruvate-producing metabolism to anaerobic lactate-producing metabolism.[51,52] DHEA administration results in a shift from the anaerobic to the more normal aerobic metabolism with a change in the pyruvate-lactate ratio and a reversion to more normal levels of lactic dehydrogenase and glycogen.[51]

Because there is less electrical energy from impaired metabolism, EEG waves in patients with organic brain syndrome generally decline in frequency and energy. The fast beta waves of cerebral cortex activity disappear, the fast alpha waves of thalamic coordination of cortical discharge decline, and the slow delta and theta waves of basic brain function continue about normally. This is possibly because some malfunction of the sodium pump in transmitting nerve impulses results in sodium entering the cell, reversing polarity, and reducing electrical activity.[52] DHEA often causes the EEG energies to return toward normal. This is especially true in experimentally treated cats and less so in people. The improvement has been attributed to the stabilization of ganglion cell metabolism. It has not been established that the EEG improvement results in clinical improvement.[6,51,54]

Cyclic AMP mediates a variety of cell responses, including peptide–amino acid hormone message transmission and some neurotransmission effects as second messengers. Cyclic AMP is catabolized by phosphodiesterase. DHEA specifically inhibits brain phosphodiesterase and, thus, allows an increase in cyclic AMP and improved efficiency of cellular performance.

ATP catabolism is inhibited by DHEA, again indicating an improved energy balance and oxygen utilization in the cell.

Elevated levels of alkaline phosphatase, indicative of some tissue malfunction, return to normal with DHEA. The increase of alkaline phosphatase correlates well with cerebral edema.

Succinic dehydrogenase, an enzyme of terminal oxidation, increases after DHEA administration, again indicating better oxygen utilization, presumably from improved neuronal activity.

As ganglion cell metabolism declines, sugars accumulate in the astrocytes, primarily around the glial processes of supportive cells. These processes become covered with a thick coat which becomes a major part of the blood-brain barrier. The nonmetabolic activity of the ganglion cell is inversely proportional to the astroglia. DHEA seems to contribute to the normalization of astrocyte metabolism: there is decreased glycolytic activity, and the accumulated polysaccharides decline in amount.

Regulation of the energy transport and energy-dependent balance of water and electrolytes between the blood and brain by DHEA results in fewer glial cells pressing against the capillaries. This presumably explains the decreased vascular resistance and increased cerebral blood flow seen with DHEA administration. In arteriosclerotic patients there is a considerable improvement in cerebral blood flow and oxygen utilization and decreased cerebrovascular resistance. No changes are observed in those with normal brain metabolism and cerebral blood flow.[51]

It has also been suggested that DHEA inhibits neuronal uptake of norepinephrine, which influences the autonomic nervous system.[54]

In organic dementia, the average cerebral blood flow is reduced to the same extent as the severity of mental impairment, and DHEA-induced reduction of cerebral circulation time corresponds to symptomatic improvement. But here we have to remember that mental impairment may be the *cause*, not the *result* of the reduced blood flow.[31,55]

A number of studies have mentioned the beneficial effects of DHEA over the entire course of a study while placebos and vasodilators have a lesser effect or level off and then decline in effect after an initial improvement, or do not result in improvement of as many symptoms[56-59]

We must also remember something else when looking at *any* of these studies. The increased attention given to the patient-subject can result in at least a temporary improvement. For instance, studies with schoolchildren have shown that regardless of their genuine ability or lack thereof, those who are "stroked" do much better than those arbitrarily relegated to the dull category and ignored. And it is a well-known phenomenon of drug studies in geriatric patients that the attention given them increases their feelings of worth and sociability.

Studies correlating cerebral blood perfusion and symptoms in 36 patients treated with DHEA over 12 months found that those with normal perfusion had improved symptoms if there were symptoms, those with borderline declines in perfusion rates had improved flow rates and symptoms, and those with poor perfusion rates had noticeably improved perfusion rates and symptoms. However the improvements in perfusion rates in the latter two categories did not bring them up to the baseline for the next less afflicted group. Again, the improved perfusion was attributed to improved neuronal activity.[52]

Aside from theory, what do studies tell us about the value of DHEA? One review of 12 trials with DHEA found significant improvement in 13 symptoms of dementia, but because the improvements were all small, the authors concluded that until further research and better methodology was available, DHEA could be considered of only minor value. They assessed 36 variables in three or more studies and grouped them under mental status, cognition, physical symptoms, daily living, personality, affect, and aggregates of all of these. There was a statistcally significant improvement in at least half of the studies. All the cognitive variables improved, but few of the physical or daily living variables did so.[59]

Other studies have either been contradictory or have given further insights. The effects of DHEA appear gradually over at least six weeks and remain. This is in contrast to placebos where there may be an initial improvement which soon wanes, or with vasodilators where the effects are more immediate but not so great in the long run. Some studies also find improvement in anorexia and headache.[60–63]

Several recommendations may be made for the most effective use of DHEA. Those with mild to moderate impairment are most suited for treatment, probably because not much irreversible damage has occurred. In one study of early Alzheimer's disease in four patients, one improved dramatically by 90 days, one improved slightly, and two did not improve at all. Those who are severely afflicted are not likely to improve much. At least 3 to 4 weeks are required for any noticeable improvement, and improvement should not be expected in all parameters. Simply halting further decline may be a valid goal.[64,65]

We have dealt at length on DHEA because its development, use, and promotion may be a forerunner of additional useful research. Certainly anything that promises to relieve the organic dementias is worthy of encouragement and support. We believe that such drugs as DHEA add to the understanding of the disease, and they may, in one form or another, eventually prove to be as great as their promise.

Increased Oxygen to the Brain

Hyperbaric Oxygen   The use of hyperbaric oxygen in elderly demented persons is based on the theory that there may be many cortical cells operating on a suboptimum oxygen supply. The cells may get enough oxygen to remain alive but not to function normally. By enhancing the oxygen available to cells, can their function be improved?

Intermittent oxygenation has significantly improved mental functioning in some patients with organic brain syndrome associated with cerebral arteriosclerosis, senile psychosis, and cerebral vascular insufficiency. In those whose dementia is not due to vascular disease and whose vasculature is normal, hyperbaric oxygenation would seem to be of little value. When brain cells are dead in chronic organic brain syndrome, there can be no benefit. However it may be of some benefit in mild hypoxia. There have been about eight rigorous studies of hyperbaric oxygenation on cognitive functioning. The positive and negative results have been about equal. Even in those with moderate to severe dementia, while the treatment has not improved the dementia, it has increased physical activity, restlessness, and aggression in elderly subjects.[66-70] Another related study found significant improvement in a few patients treated with either normobaric or hyperbaric oxygen.

Vasodilators   Many older persons with cerebral arteriosclerosis have reduced cerebral circulation and cerebral hypoxia, which can eventually reduce cerebral metabolism. The rationale for the use of cerebral vasodilators is the belief that ischemic damage to the nervous system can be relieved or prevented by increasing oxygen supply through arterial dilation.[71,72]

EEG changes follow changes in cerebral metabolism as pointed out earlier. Patients with arteriosclerotic dementia have good correlation between the declining cerebral blood flow, decreased oxygen consumption, and EEG slowing.[73] Metabolism accompanying aging may cause reduced demand for blood and mental deterioration, and not vice versa.[74] Thus cerebral vasodilation alone does not always help. Above the previously mentioned 60 mmHg, blood flow to the brain is primarily regulated by nervous tissue metabolism. Second, because arteriosclerotic vessels are less able to dilate, the dilation of all cerebral blood vessels can shunt blood away from the ischemic area and aggravate the condition. Moreover, the increased blood supply does not necessarily result in increased metabolism.[72] Third, there are not many elastic fibers in the smaller cerebral vessels. This results in their being less responsive than systemic vessels. Thus, because the resulting vasodilation may be more systemic than cerebral, there may be problems with orthostatic hypotension.[75]

Those with only minor cerebrovascular problems are most suited for *cyclandelate* therapy, as early therapy of cerebrovascular disease is important if there is to be any good done.[76] Studies in normal elderly people with only minor mental impairment have shown results which favor cyclandelate over placebos. Other studies have shown that cyclandelate may arrest the expected mental decline in those with cerebral arteriosclerosis but does not improve mentation. The drug apparently does not affect physical condition or gross behavior. Other reviews find improved orientation, behavior, and vocabulary but with no improvement in self-care, the activities of daily living, recent memory, or mood.[76-79] We have had no extensive experience with this drug. We have not noticed that any of our patients got worse when the drug was discontinued.

Papaverine also increases cerebral circulation in arteriosclerotic patients. EEG abnormalities from arteriosclerosis have improved in as many as five out of six patients along with grooming and cooperation but not memory. There seems to be least benefit in improving anxiety and depression.[71,73,80,81] Papaverine has been noted to antagonize the effects of levodopa in patients with Parkinson's disease. So it has been suggested that papaverine may be effective not only because it is a vasodilator but also because it blocks the effects of dopamine. Hence it may act similarly to other agents which block dopamine, such as haloperidol, which has also improved the affect, memory, and orientation in some geriatric patients. Our own opinion is that this action, rather than enhancing any benefits from papaverine, may detract from them. There are several reasons for this.

Increasing levels of monoamine oxidase in the aging brain, seen especially in women, lead to depression by increased catabolism of dopamine and norepinephrine. Papaverine tends to block the actions of one of these neurotransmitters even further. Demented persons already have low levels of dopamine in some of the affected brain areas. And remembering that Parkinson's disease is characterized by low levels of dopamine in the nigrostriatal pathways of the basal ganglia, some demented Parkisonian patients treated with levodopa are improved in their dementia as well as their Parkinson's disease. (However, some are worsened.) In contrast, cyclandelate, which does not block dopamine, was rated by one reviewer as superior to papaverine in improving mental function in organic brain syndrome.[83]

Whatever their actions, vasodilators are used to treat such symptoms as confusion, lack of self-care, dizziness, depression, and unsociability, which are known to be caused by cerebrovascular disease. However, vascular disease is not significant in many changes with senile dementia, and the diminished blood flow is caused by the decline in the number of functioning brain cells and the decline in metabolic activity in the remaining cells.[80] These symptoms can be caused by many other organic, psychological, and drug-induced cerebral disorders. So there is not much reasons to use cerebral vasodilators or any other drug until the cause of the syndrome is known. More studies with patients in clear diagnostic categories are needed.

In our opinion, the inconclusive results reported from the use of vasodilators does not justify their use. Rather, the attention given by nurses to dosing can be put to better use. The experimental evidence, however, is intriguing and we hope for further progress.

Anticoagulants   The rationale for using anticoagulants is the theory that either a circulatory deficiency, usually a sclerotic narrowing of the arteries supplying the brain or a sludging or thrombosing of blood in the cerebral vessels, plays a major role in the development of dementia. We do know that the sclerosis may sometimes cause dementia, but we have no idea whether sludging, the tendency of blood to thicken after passing a small lesion, plays a role in dementia.

Blood clotting may cause the mental decline in multi-infarct dementia, as mental decline sometimes occurs before motor symptoms, and at least some senile dementia may be caused by blood clotting. Thus, senile dementia may sometimes be caused by a stroke. By preventing clotting and sludging, more blood reaches the partially deprived areas to restore some lost function.

A Pittsburgh psychiatrist, using the anticoagulant dicumarol, has stopped mental deterioration and found universal improvement in elderly patients with transient ischemic attacks or recurrent strokes. He found that the mental decline stopped and started with fluctuations in prothrombin time as therapy started and stopped.[84,85]

In contrast, at least one other study using warfarin found no significant changes in the psychological variables of severely impaired or defective cognitive and mental functioning. It is interesting to note that although the warfarin-treated patients did not improve, neither did they deteriorate. An equally afflicted control group deteriorated significantly during the same period.[86]

The major hindrance to anticoagulant therapy is the adverse effects of serious bleeding in about 25 percent of those treated. There is a relatively high incidence of thromboembolic complications after stopping therapy, patients must be carefully selected and then closely supervised for adverse effects, and the effects of other drugs and there is a danger of soft infarcts in the brain.[85]

Although it is possible that coumarin anticoagulants have some effect in the brain other than their anticoagulant role, it is hard to believe there can be universal improvement. The halt in mental decline with warfarin seems a bit more plausible. This is still highly experimental and, as data is lacking, quite unproven. As with their use in cardiovascular disease, we believe that the dangers of prolonged treatment with anticoagulants outweigh the benefits.

Carbonic Anhydrase Inhibitors   These have been used for their vasodilating effects. Carbonic anhydrase catalyzes the reversible hydration of carbon dioxide, which decreases the extracellular pH, to cause cerebral vasodilation. Using one carbonic anhydrase inhibitor that passes the blood-brain barrier, it was found that there was a significant increase in cerebral blood flow in mildly demented geriatric patients but no consistent mental improvement.[87]

Symptom Supression   About half of those with senile dementia have symptoms which may be even more disabling than the brain syndrome. About 20 percent of those with Alzheimer's disease have paranoid reactions. Insight and self-evaluation are lost, as well as the ability for abstract reasoning. Because paranoid individuals initially have a good memory, the nature of the paranoid reaction may be obscure.[72,88] Later, the combinations of symptoms may become overwhelming to the patients and those who care for them. Suspicion, hostility, and dreadful hallucinations may occur before senile dementia is suspected.

People with cerebral arteriosclerosis may have similar symptoms but are more apt to have some understanding of their condition. Such understanding may be partly responsible for the profound depression in many stroke patients. In addition, many demented patients are hyperactive, agitated, irritable, hostile, untidy, or have other symptoms that require treatment.

The treatment is then directed to helping the patients to be as comfortable as possible while preventing complications. The treatment is symptomatic with no effect on the underlying disease.

The classes and drugs we are concerned with here are antipsychotics, antianxiety drugs, sedative-hypnotics, and antidepressants.

Antipsychotics It has been estimated that as many as 80 percent of the elderly demented take unnecessary tranquilizers.[90] This, of course, does not include their short-term use for such crises as the violent symptoms which sometimes occur in organic brain syndromes. Such a figure suggests that tranquilizers may be used simply to render an old person tractable, if not stupid. We have found that a stable environment and warm acceptance often make tranquilizers unnecessary. Nevertheless, drugs play an important role in allowing dear old demented people to live at their best.

Because mind-altering drugs are the most frequently used class of drugs, it seems worthwhile to reiterate part of what we said in the last chapter.

Rauwolfia products. These drugs are seldom used because of their hypotensive and depressing effects and the fact that they have lower efficacy than other antipsychotics.

Butyrophenones. The prototype of these drugs is haloperidol (Haldol). Butyrophenones have some ability to control agitation and hyperactivity, but also cause a high incidence of extrapyramidal reactions. They are useful in controlling hallucinations and have less tendency to put a person to sleep than other antipsychotic drugs.

Thioxanthenes. Drugs such as thiothixene (Navane) and chlorprothixene (Taractan) are relatively new drugs which are being used more and more. Thiothixene does not seem particularly useful in chronic organic brain syndrome, often being no better than a placebo. Fortunately it seems safe, and its side effects are few and mild.[91-93]

Phenothiazines. This group of drugs probably has done more to revolutionize the care of psychotic patients than any other factor. As with any class of drugs, the best one may be the one with which the physician is most familiar. He or she will then know what to expect, will watch for untoward effects, and will check for symptoms of overdosing or underdosing. Although one does not seem to be much better than another, thioridazine (Mellaril) and acetophenazine (Tindal) seem to be the most widely used phenothiazines in older patients. They may all cause confusion, wandering about, and a stereotyped behavior in larger doses.[83,94]

Several studies have produced conflicting data on *Mesoridazine (Serentil)*. Some have found it to be of little value. Others have found it most valuable in those patients whose organic brain syndromes present with prominent hostility and psychomotor excitement. In these patients, the agitation, irritability, hostility, poor impulse control, and paranoid ideas respond well, and there may be some improvement in depression. As with all other drugs in this class, large doses cause oversedation or increased retardation.[95-97]

The drug *chlorpromazine (Thorazine)* is most useful in patients who are very agitated, combative, and hyperactive. However, its tendency to cause drowsiness and dizziness can be particularly dangerous to the ambulatory geriatric patient. There is a greater incidence of parkinsonian reactions such as tremors, weakness, and rigidity than with other phenothiazines. There are also pronounced cardiac and hepatic effects.[90]

Our drug of choice is *thioridazine (Mellaril)*. It is helpful in agitation. Unlike certain others in this group, it does not often bring on or aggravate depression. It will frequently calm a violent person without rendering him stupid or immobile. It may occasionally cause low blood pressure or undesired anticholinergic effects. It is not as sedating as chlorpromazine and causes fewer extrapyramidal symptoms. Nonspecific ECG abnormalities resembling hypokalemia are frequent, but are reversed upon administration of potassium. In any event, they seem of little consequence.[98]

All the phenothiazines may cause hypotension, a particularly dangerous situation, especially if there is also cerebrovascular insufficiency. There is increased potential for toxic confusion in organic brain syndrome, and even a small dose may increase confusion and mental impairment.[89]

Antianxiety Drugs   *Diazepam* (Valium) and *clorazepate* (Tranxene) may be useful in tense and anxious patients who are not agitated or confused. Higher doses, paradoxically, have increased agitation, aggression, and irritability. They sometimes impair thinking and cause ataxia and weakness. Anxiety and depression generally respond better to thioridazine.[99]

Sedative-hypnotics   The sleep disturbances that appear in organic brain syndrome are both common and hard to manage. Insomnia or reversed sleep patterns may appear, so that the person dozes throughout the day and becomes restless at night. This is the "sundown syndrome."

Slow-acting *barbiturates* such as butabarbital (Butisol) are safe and effective in moderate doses, but all of the barbiturates may decrease further an already marginal cerebral metabolism so that agitation and confusion may be worsened in an old patient with organic brain syndrome.

One novel approach to treating the "sundown syndrome" is to give coffee at bedtime. Although anecdotal reports of the efficacy of this are available, one study found that only three out of twelve patients slept better.[100]

Alternatives to drugs include keeping patients awake and active during the day. This makes more sense than allowing them to sleep during the day and giving them sleeping pills at night.[101]

Antidepressants   A common disturbance associated with organic brain syndrome is depression, characterized by anger, resentment, and noisy wandering about.

The confusion seen in organic brain syndrome does not affect all the spheres of consciousness. Even when severely confused, people may well appreciate their physical and mental losses and become quite depressed. This depression in turn worsens the already present organic deficits.[102]

Some of the previously mentioned drugs may also act as antidepressants. For instance, thioridazine and diazepam may help agitated depression better than a tricyclic antidepressant.

Tricyclic antidepressants. These drugs are useful in treating the depression associated with organic brain syndrome. They all act in the same basic manner although there is some difference in their specific effects in the reuptake of norepinephrine or serotonin at synaptic junctions.

Monoamine oxidase inhibitors. Let's look at some of the warnings and contraindications for the MAO inhibitors, and then we can think about their uses in treating depression. Because the most serious side effects involve changes in blood pressure, it is not advisable to use these drugs in elderly or debilitated persons or where there is hypertension or cardiovascular or cerebrovascular disease. There may be hypertensive crises if the person is also taking sympathomimetics, methyldopa, levodopa, or tricyclic antidepressants. Furthermore, they should not be used if renal function is impaired. Side effects include insomnia, constipation, anorexia, nausea, vomiting, dry mouth, urinary retention, drowsiness, orthostatic hypotension, weakness, and peripheral edema. The package insert for Parnate (tranylcypromine) states that it should not be used in patients over 60 years of age or who are taking antihypertensive drugs or diuretics. Package inserts for other such drugs also warn against their use in elderly or debilitated patients. Rather obviously, MAO inhibitors are only useful if all other therapy fails, and the person is young, otherwise healthy, and takes no other drugs.

Stimulants. From time immemorial, stimulants have been used to increase energy, overcome depression, and improve memory, motivation, and attention. Strychnine, caffeine, amphetamines and methylphenidate (Ritalin), and others have been used to make people feel better. Of the group, only caffeine, as in coffee, and methylphenidate have a place in geriatric practice. Generally stimulants are useless if not actually harmful. They may cause convulsions, increased heart work, anorexia, irritability, restlessness, and insomnia. Coffee, even if decaffeinated, is useful because it is tasty and rich in potassium.

Miscellaneous

Procaine HCl. For at least 20 years sporadic reports have come from Europe extolling the rejuvenating properties of acidified procaine injections. Repeated studies in the United States have failed to show any benefit in demented patients.[104] Fortunately, it also seems harmless. It does cause one to wonder about the differences between old Rumanians and old Americans.

Folic acid. One report cites a folate deficiency in a demented patient. Upon treating the folate deficiency, the dementia improved. The investigator suggested that the sleeplessness, forgetfulness, irritability, confusion, and slow mental deterioration in some chronic schizophrenics may be due to a prolonged folate deficiency. In this respect it is interesting to note that drugs known to lower serum folate levels include barbiturates, phenytoin and primidone, phenyl-butazone, nitrofurantoin, alcohol, some analgesics, and possibly phenothiazines (Mellaril, Thorazine, Compazine, Phenergan).[105,106]

Another elderly demented person treated with vitamin B_{12} and folic acid had a rapid return to intellectual and behavioral normality but with amnesia for the period of psychosis and dementia.[107]

It is interesting to speculate on the extent to which the above-named drugs and nutritional deficiencies may contribute to these syndromes.

SUMMARY

We have gone into a good bit of theory in this chapter because we believe that changes in the central nervous system are the hallmarks of aging itself. The sheer number of disturbed old people warrants a discussion like this. The sheer number of psychotropic drugs, the most frequently prescribed of all drugs, requires lengthy treatment.

We see that there are many treatments aimed at the causes of dementia. Each has its theoretical and physiological underpinnings and rationale. Although none is universally effective for all symptoms or all patients, a number have provided varying degrees of improvement in some symptoms in certain patients. A number of studies note that although patients did not improve, neither did they decline with a disease characterized by the steady deterioration of the patient.

More studies are needed in which patients are placed into clear diagnostic categories, such as Alzheimer's disease, multi-infarct dementia, cerebrovascular dementia, and mixtures of these. We must learn more about the long-term effects of many of these drugs. We must remember that it is impossible to return the more severely afflicted patients to normal mental function. When a brain cell is dead, it is permanently dead. But if the decline can be slowed or halted, or if life can be made more tolerable and enjoyable, even for those caring for the patients, and especially if there is a little improvement in any function even for a short time, we are doing well.

We are frequently impressed by how well some demented patients do. Many are charming, kind, and loving. All are worthy of our best thoughts and efforts.

Besides drugs and purely custodial care, there are other forms of therapy. Not all are equally applicable to dementia, and all are variations on a theme.

We now turn to Parkinson's disease.

REFERENCES

1 Ronald W., Angel, "Understanding and Diagnosing Senile Dementia," *Geriatrics* **32**:47–49(1977).
2 H. S. Wang and E. W. Busse, "Dementia in Old Age," in C. E. Wells (ed.), *Dementia*, Davis, Philadelphia, 1971, p. 152.

3   Robert Katzman, "The Prevalence and Malignancy of Alzheimer's Disease. A Major Killer," *Arch. Neurol* **33**:217–218(1976).

4   H. S. Wang, "Dementia in Old Age," in Smith and Kinsbourne (eds.), *Aging and Dementia*, Spectrum, New York, 1977, p. 18.

5   A. J. Finestone and F. J. Bianco, "Organic Brain Syndrome," *Am. Fam. Physician* **6**:74(1977).

6   J. Roubicek et al., "An Ergot Alkaloid Preparation (Hydergine) in Geriatric Therapy," *J. Amer. Geriatr. Soc.* **20**:222–229,(1972).

7   Mary R. Andriola, "Role of E.E.G. in Evaluating Central Nervous System Dysfunction," *Geriatrics* **33**:59–65(1978).

8   V. Marks, "Spontaneous Hypoglycemia," *Hospital Medicine* **1**:118–125(1966).

9   T. G. Judge, "Hypokalemia in the Elderly," *Gerontol. Clin.* **10**:102(1968).

10   S. Strandgaard et al., "Autoregulation of Brain Evaluation in Severe Arterial Hypertension," *Br. Med. J.* **1**:507–510(1973).

11   Robert S. Schwab, "Treatment of Parkinson's Disease in the Aged," *J. Am. Geriatr. Soc.* **4**:491–497(1956).

12   Robert S. Schwab, "Problems in the Treatment of Parkinson's Disease in Elderly Patients," *Geriatrics* **14**:545–558(1959).

13   Bernard Grad et al., "Effects of Levodopa Therapy in Patients with Parkinson's Disease: Statistical Evidence for Reduced Tolerance to Levodopa in the Elderly," *J. Am. Geriatr. Soc.* **22**:489–493(1974).

14   C. Powell, "The Use and Abuse of Drugs in Brain Failure," *Age and Aging*, Supplement to **6**:83(1977).

15   B. M. Learoyd, "Psychotropic Drugs and the Elderly Patient," *Med. J. Aust.* **1**:1131(1972).

16   Gaston P. DeLemos et al., "Effects of Diazepam Suspension in Geriatric Patients Hospitalized for Psychiatric Illness," *J. Am. Geriatr. Soc.* **13**:355–359(1965).

17   Carl Salzman et al., "Psychopharmacologic Investigations in Elderly Volunteers: Effect of Diazepam in Males," *J. Am. Geriatr. Soc.* **23**:451–457(1975).

18   James K. Martilla et al., "Potential Untoward Effects of Long-Term use of Flurazepam in Geriatric Patients," *J. Am. Pharm. Assoc.* **NS17**:692–695(1977).

19   D. J. Greenblatt et al., "Flurazepam HC1: A Benzodiazepine Hypnotic" *Ann. Intern. Med.* **83**:237(1975).

20   Keith Dawson-Butterwort, "The Chemopsychotherapeutics of Geriatric Sedation," *J. Am. Geriatr. Soc.* **18**:97–114(1970).

21   Leslie S. Libow, "Pseudosenility: Acute and Reversible Organic Brain Syndromes," *J. Am. Geriatr. Soc.* **21**:112–120(1973).

22   B. J. Gurland, "The Comparative Frequency of Depression in Various Adult Age Groups," *J. Gerontol.* **31**:283(1976).

23   M. A. Lipton, "Age Differentiation in Depression: Biochemical Aspects," *J. Gerontol.* **31**:293(1976).

24   W. G. Vogel et al., "Endogenous Depression Improvement and Rapid Eye Movement Pressure," *Arch. Gen. Psychiatry* **34**:96(1977).

25   S. Cath, "Beyond Depression-The Depleted State," *Can. Psychiatr. Assoc. J.*, Special Supplement to **11**:5329(1966).

26   S. Cath, "Individual Adaptation in the Middle Years," *J. Geriatr. Psychiatry* **9**:19(1976).

27 H. Graves, "Depression in the Aged: Theoretical Concepts," *J. Am. Geriatr. Soc.* **25**:447–449(1977).

28 W. J. Dekininck et al., "Cerebral Vasoreactivity in Senile Dementia," *Gerontology* **23**:148–160(1977).

29 D. Simard et al., "Regional Cerebral Blood Flow and its Regulation in Dementia," *Brain* **94**:273–288(1971).

30 Seymour Kety, "Human Cerebral Blood Flow and Oxygen Consumption as Related to Aging," *Res. publ.* **35**:31–49(1956).

31 Walter D. Obrist, "Regional Cerebral Blood Flow in Senile and Presenile Dementia," *Neurology* **20**:315–322(1970).

32 B. Falck et al, *Scand. J. Clin. Lab. Invest.* 1968 22Suppl. 102 page Vi:B

33 Saul Kent, "Alzheimer's Disease, Senile Dementia, and Related Disorders" in "N.I.H. Workshop, Classifying and Treating Organic Brain Syndromes," *Geriatrics:* **32**:87–95(1977).

34 P. Davies et al., "Selective Loss of Central Cholinergic Neurons in Alzheimer's Disease," *Lancet* **ii**:1403(1976).

35 Bowen, et al "Neurotransmitter-Related Enzymes and Indices of Hypoxia in Senile Dementia and other Abiotrophies," *Brain* **99**:459–496(1976).

36 Tomlinson et al., "Observations on the Brains of Non-demented old People," *J. Neurol. Sci.* **7**:331–356(1968).

37 J. A. N. Corsellis, *Mental Illness and the Aging Brain, Oxford, London, 1962.*

38 W. D. Obrist, "Cerebral Physiology of the Aged. Influence of Circulatory Disorders," in C. M. Gaitz (ed.), *Aging and the Brain* Plenum, New York, 19??, pp. 117–133.

39 Smith and Kinsbourne, *"Vascular Disease and Dementia in the Elderly,"* in Smith and Kinsbourne (eds.), *Aging and Dementia,* Spectrum, New York, 1977.

40 Anon., "Drugs for Improvement of Cerebral Function in the Elderly" *Medical Letter* **18**(9):38—39(1976).

41 S. Munch-Petersen et al., "RNA Treatment of Dementia: A Double Blind Study," *Acta Neurol. Scand.* **50**:553–572(1974).

42 D. E. Cameron and L. Solyom, "Effects of Ribonucleic Acid on Memory," *Geriatrics* **16**:74–81(1961).

43 D. E. Cameron et al., "Effects of Ribonucleic Acid on Memory Defects in the Aged," *Am. J. Psychiatry* **120**:320–325(1962).

44 David A. Drachman and Steven Stahl, "Extrapyramidal Dementia and Levodopa," *Lancet* **i**:809(1975).

45 Gerald A. Broe and F. I. Caird, "Levodopa for Parkinsonism in Elderly and Demented Patients," *Med. J. Aust.* **i**:630–635(1973).

46 John Pearce and Iris Pearce, "Parkinsonism and Dementia: Effects of Levodopa," *Lancet* **i**:1245(1975).

47 A. H. Rajput and B. Rozdilsey, "Parkinsonism and Dementia: Effects of Levodopa," *Lancet* **i**:1084(1975).

48 Manuel. Riklen, "An L-DOPA Paradox: Bipolar Behavioral Alterations," *J. Am. Geriatr. Soc.* **20**:572–575(1972).

49 John Stirling Meyer et al., "Neurotransmitter Precursor Amino Acids in the Treatment of Multi-infarct Dementia and Alzheimer's Disease," *J. Am. Geriatr. Soc.* **25**:289–298(1977).

50 Dunner and Goodwin, "Effect of L-Tryptophan on Brain Serotonin Metabolism in Depressed Patients," *Arch. Gen. Psychiatry* **26**:364(1972).

51 H. Emmenegger and W. Meier-Ruge, "The Actions of Hydergine on the Brain," *Pharmacology* **1**:65–78(1968).

52 B. Mongeau, "The Effects of Hydergine on the Transit Time of Cerebral Circulation in Diffuse Cerebral Insufficiency," *Eur. J. Clin. Pharmacol.* **7**(3):169–175(1974).

53 R. Dixon et al., "Experimental Cerebral Insufficiency," Scientific Exhibit, Federation of American Societies for Experimental Biology, 57th Annual Meeting, 1973.

54 W. Pacha and R. Salzman, "Inhibition of the Re-uptake of Neuronally Liberated Noradrenalin and Receptor Blocking Action of some Ergot Alkaloids," *Br. J. Pharmacol.* **38**:439(1970).

55 C. C. McHenry et al., "Hydergine Effect on Cerebral Circulation in Cerebrovascular Disease," *J. Neurol. Sci.* **13**:475(1971).

56 Albert J. Bazo, "An Ergot Alkaloid Preparation (Hydergine) versus Papaverine in Treating Common Complaints of the Aged: Double Blind Study," *J. Am. Geriatr. Soc.* **21**:63–71(1973).

57 Herbert J. Rosen, "Mental Decline in the Elderly: Pharmacotherapy (Ergot Alkaloids versus Papaverine)," *J. Am. Geriatr. Soc.* **23**:169–174(1975).

58 Jere Nelson, "Relieving Select Symptoms of the Elderly," *Geriatrics* **30**:133–142(1975).

59 John. R. Hughes et al., "An Ergot Alkaloid Preparation (Hydergine) in the Treatment of Dementia: Critical Review of the Clinical Literature," *J. Am. Geriatr. Soc.* **24**:490–497(1976).

60 B. J. Wilder and E. F. Gonyer, "The Effects of the Dihydrogenated Ergot Alkaloids on Symptoms of Aging" Scientific Exhibit, A. M. A. Convention, New York, New York, 1973.

61 Morris Ditch et al., "An Ergot Preparation (Hydergine) in the Treatment of Cerebrovascular Disorders in the Geriatric Patient: Double Blind Study," *J. Am. Geriatr. Soc.* **19**:208–217(1971).

62 David M. Baben, "An Ergot Alkaloid Preparation (Hydergine) for Relief of Symptoms of Cerebrovascular Insufficiency," *J. Am. Geriatr. Soc.* **20**:22–24(1972).

63 F. Triboletti and H. Ferri, "Hydergine for Treatment of Symptoms of Cerebrovascular Insufficiency," *Curr. Ther. Res.* **11**:609–620(1969).

64 Ernst Burian, "An Ergot Alkaloid Preparation (Hydergine) in the Treatment of Presenile Brain Atrophy (Alzheimer's Disease): Case Report" *J. Am. Geriatr. Soc.* **22**:126–128(1974).

65 Anon., "Hydergine: General Summary of Information," Sandoz Publications, 1976.

66 Larry W. Thompson et al., "Effects of Hyperbaric Oxygen on Behavioral and Physiological Measures in Elderly Demented Patients," *J. Gerontol.* **31**(1):23–28(1976).

67 Eleanor A. Jacobs et al., "Hyperoxygenation: A Central Nervous System Activator," *J. Geriatr. Psychiatry:* **5**:107–136(1972).

68 Alvin I. Goldfarb, "Hyperbaric Oxygen Treatment of Organic Mental Syndrome in Aged Persons," *J. Gerontol.* **27**:212–217(1972).

69 Eleanor A. Jacobs et al., "Hyperoxygenation Effect on Cognitive Functioning in the Aged," *N. Engl. J. Med.* **281**:753–757(1969).

70 D. K. Dastor et al., "Effects of Aging on Cerebral Circulation and Metabolism in Man," in J. E. Birren et al. (eds.), *Human Aging: A Biological and Behavioral Study* U.S.P.H.S. Publication #986, Washington, D.C. pp 59–76.

71   Francis H. Stern, "Management of Chronic Brain Syndrome Secondary to Cerebral Arteriosclerosis, with Special Reference to Papaverine Hydrochloride," *J. Am. Geriatr. Soc.* **18**:507(1970).

72   Anon., "Cerebral Vasodilators," *Br. Med. J.* **ii**:702–703(1971).

73   Antonia Culebras, "Effect of Papaverine on Cerebral Electrogenesis," *Neurology* **26**:673–679(1976).

74   N. A. Lassen, "Cerebral Blood Flow and Oxygen Consumption," *Physiol. Rev.* **39**:183(1959).

75   V. Ronnoc-Jessen, "Cerebral Complications in Nitroglycerin Treatment of Angina Pectoris," *Acta Med. Scand.* **174**:523–527(1963).

76   T. G. Judge, "Cyclandelate and Mental Functions: A Double Blind Cross-Over Trial in Normal Elderly Subjects," *Age and Aging* **2**:121(1973).

77   Peter Hall, "Cyclandelate in the Treatment of Cerebral Arteriosclerosis," *J. Am. Geriatr. Soc.* **24**:41(1976).

78   John. Young et al., "Treatment of Cerebral Manifestations of Arteriosclerosis with Cyclandelate," *Br. J. Psychiatry* **124**:177–180(1974).

79   Anon., "Drugs for Dementia" *Drug and Therapeutics Bulletin* **13**(22):85(1975).

80   von B. Huenermann, R. Felix et al., "On the Action of Papaverine Hydrochloride on Cerebral Circulation: Studies with a Scintillation Camera-Computer System" *Arzneimittel Forsch.* **25**(4):652–653(1975).

81   Loretta M. McQuillen et al., "Evaluation of E.E.G. and Clinical Changes Associated with Pavabid Therapy in Chronic Brain Syndrome," *Curr. Ther. Res.* **16**:49–58(1974).

82   Roland J. Branconnier and Jonathen Cole, "Effects of Chronic Papaverine Administration on Mild Senile Organic Brain Syndrome," *J. Am. Geriatr. Soc.* **25**:458–459(1977).

83   Thomas A. Ban, "Psychopathology, Psychopharmacology, and the Organic Brain Sundromes," *Psychosomatics*.

84   Arthur C. Walsh, "Arterial Insufficiency of the Brain: Progression Prevented by Long-term Anticoagulant Therapy in Eleven Patients," *J. Am. Geriatr. Soc.* **17**:93–104(1969).

85   Arthur C. Walsh, "Prevention of Senile and Presenile Dementia by Bishydroxycoumarin (Dicumarol) Therapy," *J. Am. Geriatr. Soc.* **17**:477–487(1965).

86   Jack Ratner et al., "Anticoagulant Therapy for Senile Dementia," *J. Am. Geriatr. Soc.* **20**:556–559(1972).

87   D. J. Wyper, "Effects of a Carbonic Anhydrase Inhibitor on Cerebral Blood Flow in Geriatric Patients," *J. Neurol. Neurosurg. Psychiatry* **39**:885–889(1976).

88   Whanger "Paranoid Symptoms in the Senium," in Eisdorfer and Fann (eds.), *Psychopharmacology and Aging, Advances in Behavioral Biology,* Plenum Press, New York, 1972.

89   Robert F. Prien, "Chemotherapy in Chronic Organic Brain Syndrome- A Review of the Literature," *Psychopharmacol. Bull.* **9**(4):5–20(1973).

90   Jacob D. Hoogerbeets and John LaWall, "Changing Concepts of Psychiatric Problems in the Aged," *Geriatrics* **30**:83–87(1975).

91   D. P. Birkett et al., "Thiothixene in the Treatment of Diseases of the Senium" *Curr. Ther. Res.* **14**(12):775–779(1972).

92   Richard T. Rada and Robert Kellner, "The Effects of Thiothixene in Geriatric

Patients with Chronic Brain Syndrome," *Psychopharmacol. Bull.* **12**(2):30–32(1976).

93 Richard T. Rada and Robert Kellner, "Thiothixene in the Treatment of Chronic Organic Brain Syndrome," *J. Am. Geriatr. Soc.* **24**:105–107(1976).

94 L. A. Cahn and H. F. A. Diesfeldt, "The Use of Neuroleptics in the Treatment of Dementia in Old Age," *Psychiat. Neurol. Neurochir (Amst.)* **76**:411–420(1973).

95 Stanley Goldstein, "The Use of Mesoridazine in Geriatrics," *Curr. Ther. Res.* **16**:316–323(1974).

96 Burton Goldstein and Walter Dippy, "A Clinical Evaluation of Mesoridazine (Serentil) in Geriatric Patients," *Curr. Ther. Res.* **9**:256–260(1967).

97 Anon., "Serentil for Chronic Brain Syndrome," *Med. Lett. Drugs Ther.* **17**(16):68(1968).

98 David J. Greenblatt and Richard I. Shader, "Rational Use of Psychotropic Drugs: III Major Tranquilizers," *Am. J. Hosp. Pharm.* **31**:1226–1231(1974).

99 Joe S. Covington, "Alleviating Agitation, Apprehension, and Related Symptoms in Geriatric Patients A Double Blind Comparison of Phenothiazine and a Benzodiazepine," *South. Med. J.* **68**:719–724(1975).

100 Roy Ginsburg and Michael Weintraub, "Caffeine in the 'Sundown Syndrome': Report of a Negative Report".

101 B. Stotsky, "Use of Psychopharmacological Agents Among Geriatric Patients," *Clinical Handbook of Psychopharmacology* edited by A. DiMascio and R. Shader, Basic Sciences, New York, 1970.

102 L. D. Hamilton "Antidepressant Drugs and the Organic Brain Syndromes," *Clin, Med.* **73**:49(1966).

103 Burton C. Einspruch, "Helping to Make the Final Years Meaningful for the Elderly Residents of Nursing Homes," *Dis. Nerv. Syst.* **37**(8)439–442(1976).

104 Israel Zwerling, "Effects of a Procaine Preparation (Gerovitsl H3) in Hospitalized Elderly Patients: A Double Blind Study," *J. Am. Geriatr. Soc.* **23**:355–359(1975).

105 R. W. Strachan, "Dementia and Folate Deficiency," *Q. J. Med.* **36**:189(1967).

106 J. Kariks and S. W. Perry, "Folic Acid Deficiency in Psychiatric Patients," *Med. J. Aust.* **i**:1192(1970).

107 Douglas Vann, "Vitamin B-12, Folic Acid, and the Care of Mentally Disturbed Aged Patients," *Med. J. Aust.* **ii**:1149(1972).

Chapter 10

Disorders of Motion

Disorders of motion disable more old people than any other set of symptoms. Rheumatism, arthritis, fractures, strokes, and a number of neurological disorders do their harm by hindering people from getting about. Much of rehabilitation effort goes into trying to help patients move without accidents. Disorders of motion go by several terms, which are generally understood by health workers.

Chorea Continual, purposeless, clumsy motion. Huntington's disease and Saint Vitus' dance are forms of chorea. Patients with chorea may have normal strength but be unable to feed themselves because of uncontrollable jerking of arms, head, or other parts.

Athetosis or **athetoid movement** Rhythmical, repetitive motions of extremities or face. The movements of the hands suggest those of a Hindu dancer. The face may repetitively go through a cycle of grimacing, smiling, and repose, none of which reflect emotion. Athetoid movements nearly always occur in people who are spastic, with muscles held tightly, as in cerebral palsy.

Tremors Trembling motions which occur most often in the hands but also in the head, lips, tongue, or jaw. Tremors vary in severity from person to person, and in the same person from time to time. Some tremors run in families and are not necessarily disabling; others are severe and interfere with self-care such as eating and keeping tidy. Tremors are usually accompanied by stiffness.

Paralysis   The inability to move because of failure of the nervous system to transmit or receive impulses. Paralysis may be spastic, with muscles held rigid, or flaccid, with muscles relaxed.

Paresis   Partial paralysis; generally considered a weakness of one or more muscle groups.

Dystonia   Disordered tone of muscles in which they don't contract and relax in sequence to allow appropriate posture or locomotion. Dystonia may be so severe as to cause grotesque posture or deformity.

Tics   Jerky, repetitive motions that may be voluntary, such as a simple nervous habit, or may accompany other disorders.

Twitches   Particularly about the eyelids, may be entirely benign, but twitches due to muscle fibrillation may indicate serious neurological disease.

Ataxia   A lack of muscular coordination due to a loss of proprioception or position sense. People with ataxia may fall simply because they lose awareness of where their feet are placed.

Akathisia   A state of pronounced restlessness in which a person finds it difficult to sit or lie quietly. In this condition movement is well coordinated and unrelieved. For example, a person may walk constantly, cross and uncross legs continually, or roll in bed so that sleep is impaired.

Akinesia   The absence or poverty of purposeful movements as seen in Parkinson's disease, in which animation of the facial muscles is lost, resulting in the classic masklike facial expression. It also refers to the loss of coordinated movement such as the normal armswing when a person walks.

Dyskinesia   Literally means disordered movement such as tardive dyskinesia, which we talked about in the last chapter. Parkinson's disease is an example of disordered movement.

PARKINSON'S DISEASE

While there are many disorders of motion, we shall devote most of this chapter to Parkinson's disease for the following reasons:

1   It is frequent and often severe among elderly people. Over a million people at any one time are afflicted with this disease.

2   It can often be helped by drugs.

3   Its symptoms are often produced by psychotropic drugs.

4   Some understanding of disordered movement has come from research in Parkinson's disease.

Parkinson's disease, then, is a example of diseases of disordered motion.

The disease was described in 1817 by Dr. James Parkinson, who called it paralysis agitans. His description follows:

Involuntary tremulous motion, with lessened muscular power, in parts not in action and even when supported; with a propensity to bend the trunk forward, and to pass from a walking to a running pace, the senses and intellects being uninjured.[1]

The term *Parkinson's disease* is confined to the original condition of unknown cause described by Parkinson. *Parkinsonism* or *Parkinson's syndrome* are terms used to describe symptoms that are similar or identical to those in Parkinson's disease. Such symptoms may be caused by drugs or by an infection, as occurred in thousands of people soon after World War I. Parkinsonism may occur as a result of or in combination with chronic brain syndrome or cerebral arteriosclerosis.

Levodopa

Much of our understanding of Parkinson's disease came in a roundabout way. Reserpine was among the first psychoactive drugs. It helped many psychotic patients, but its use produced parkinsonism in some. Eventually researchers demonstrated that reserpine depleted stores of dopamine precursors in the brain. The aim of treatment was to restore by medication the deficiency of dopamine. Dopamine, it was found, could not be transported across the membranes of brain cells. Cotzias, in 1967, found that levodopa, a precursor of dopamine, could penetrate the blood-brain barrier and that it was helpful in 8 of the 16 patients on whom he tried it.[2] Levodopa was approved for general distribution by prescription in 1970. Since then, thousands of people with Parkinson's disease have been helped, many of them dramatically.

Levodopa, though, presents a dilemma; its harmful effects may be greater than its benefits. It may itself cause dyskinesias even as it helps general mobility. Severe nausea and vomiting may preclude its use. Confusion, hallucinations, and disorientation occasionally occur. Postural hypotension with falls and faints are a risk of treatment. Levodopa may have an on-and-off effect, in which the symptoms abruptly become worse unpredictably even though the dosage remains the same. Such effects may be due to fluctuations in the concentration of levodopa in the bloodstream. Then, too, some patients apparently become refractory to levodopa after several years of treatment.

The undesirable effects of levodopa have been ascribed to its transformation to dopamine peripherally, that is, outside of the central nervous system. This hypothesis explains why such large doses of levodopa, up to 3 grams a day, must be given to overcome the blood-brain barrier. This transformation to dopamine outside the brain is responsible for much of the mischief which can be done by levodopa.

In an effort to overcome the mischievous effects, attention has been directed to inhibiting the peripheral conversion. This is done by blocking the action of dopa decarboxylase, an enzyme essential to the conversion process. Two such blockers (inhibitors) are carbidopa and benzerazide. When these inhibitors are given in conjunction with levodopa, the dose of the latter can be reduced markedly because a larger proportion of it remains in the blood stream and thus is available for conversion to dopamine in the brain. The accompanying diagram (Figure 10-1) schematically portrays the interations of levodopa, dopamine, and carbidopa.

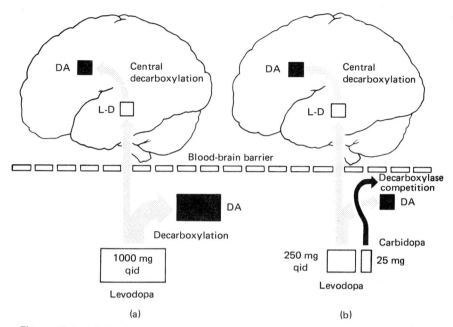

Figure 10-1 (a) A schematic representation of a therapeutic dose of levodopa as it is metabolized by dopamine, the neurotransmitter deficient in Parkinson's disease. Note that a major portion of levodopa is decarboxylated by the ring outside the blood-brain barrier. Since dopamine does not cross the blood-brain barrier, large amounts of levodopa are required to achieve therapeutic levels of dopamine in the brain. (b) A reduced quantity of levodopa is required to achieve therapeutic levels of dopamine in the brain when it is administered in conjunction with carbidopa. Carbidopa is a dopa-decarboxylase inhibitor that does not cross the blood brain barrier. *(From American Family Practice. Used with permission.)*

Because most of our patients have cardiovascular, neurological, psychiatric, or gastrointestinal problems, we seldom start treatment with levodopa alone or in its combinations with carbidopa and benzerazide, sold under the trade names of Sinemet and Madopar, respectively. If, however, an old person is getting along well taking levodopa alone or in combination, we certainly would continue to prescribe it.

The understanding of Parkinson's disease, as incomplete as it is, has helped in the understanding of other movement disorders. Huntington's disease, which is marked by progressive mental deterioration and chorea, is believed to be due to impaired dopamine metabolism, although no treatment has proved to be effective.

Anticholinergics

Coordinated movement, it is postulated, depends on a proper balance of the two neurotransmitters dopamine and acetylcholine. Simply put, dopamine initiates movement and acetylcholine sustains it. Thus, there are reports of choline in food, a precursor of acetylcholine, occasionally helping patients with certain movement disorders.

Observations on drug reactions have given support to the idea of a dopamine-acetylcholine control of movement. It has been known for over a century that anticholinergic drugs such as atropine, belladonna, and stramonium frequently relieve some of the stiffness and tremors of Parkinson's disease. Later, synthetic anticholinergic drugs were found to be helpful both in Parkinson's disease and in parkinsonism due to other causes.

A number of synthetic anticholinergic drugs may relieve parkinsonism. Among these are, by trade name, Cogentin, Artane, Akineton, Pagitane, and Kemadrin. We have had greatest experience with Cogentin and Artane. Since these drugs are relatively free of unpleasant side effects, we recommend their use. Cogentin may, however, cause drowsiness. Artane may cause constipation and excessive dryness of the mouth.

Figure 10-2 portrays normal movement (eukinesis) as a balance between acetylcholine and dopamine and demonstrates how the balance may be altered by disease and its treatment.

Other Treatments for Parkinsonism

Antihistamines such as Benadryl and Phenoxine have been useful in treatment of parkinsonism for reasons not well understood.

Somewhat paradoxically, promethazine (Phenergan), a phenothiazine drug, is occasionally helpful in Parkinson's disease. The paradox is that other phenothiazine drugs may actually produce parkinsonism.

In addition, amantadine, an antiviral agent, has found use in treating parkinsonism. It may be superior to the anticholinergic drugs but its effectiveness tends to diminish after prolonged use.

OTHER MOVEMENT DISORDERS

Parkinsonism and other disturbances of motion are often caused by drugs, especially phenothiazines, tricyclic antidepressants, and other antipsychotic drugs such as Haldol. All the phenothiazines can reduce spontaneous motor activity, and some can cause dystonias, parkinsonism, or akathisia.

In view of abnormal movement somehow being related to an imbalance of dopamine and acetylcholine, it is interesting to note that many frequently prescribed antipsychotic drugs block the action of dopamine. In our experience, parkinsonism, akathisia, and dyskinesias are the movement disorders most apt to occur as a result of medication. In many large nursing facilities there are old people with a history of mental disease. Such patients may have coped for years by taking an antipsychotic drug or tranquilizer. Thus, one can see people with blank expressions, tremors, restlessness, and muscle jerks. As mentioned earlier, tardive dyskinesia, when well established, tends to be permanent.

Because there are other drugs that do a good job in relieving nausea or promoting tranquillity, we don't believe the use of the phenothiazine Compazine is justified. We have seen truly frightful dystonia result from its use, with

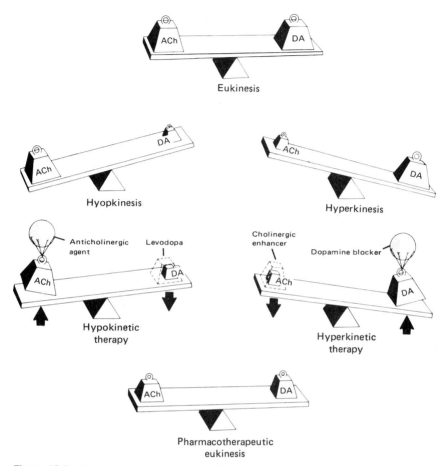

Figure 10-2 A schematic representation of the reciprocal balance between dopaminergic and cholinergic neurotransmitter systems in the basal ganglia (top diagram) resulting in eukinesis. The two diagrams on the left show the imbalance in these systems that may result in parkinsonism (upper) and the possible therapeutic interventions that counterbalance this hypokinetic state (lower). The two diagrams on the right represent the corresponding imbalance that may result in choreiform movements (upper) and the therapeutic counterbalance to these hyperkinetic disorders (lower). The eukinetic therapeutic goal in each affliction is shown in the bottom diagram. *(From American Family Practice. Used with permission.)*

grotesque jerking of head, neck, and jaw. Fortunately, most reactions to this drug are temporary.

Occasionally, centrally acting muscle relaxants may help in movement disorders. Most of them cause sedation, which may or may not be an advantage to a particular patient. More often the relaxants are used for muscle strains, sprains, and pulls. Among the relaxants are Robaxin, Norflex, Parafon, Soma, and Skelaxin.

Dantrolene has a direct relaxing effect on skeletal muscles. If a person is unable to relax spastic muscles, dantrolene may be worth a try, particularly since it seems to be relatively free of serious side effects. It is a relatively new drug and patients who take it should be observed closely for liver damage.

No discussion of movement disorders would be complete without mention of myasthenia gravis, a potentially serious, treatable, intermittent paralysis. Its understanding is linked to the understanding of other movement disorders.

In Chapter 4, acetylcholine was mentioned as a neurotransmitter. In addition to working at autonomic ganglia and visceral end organs, it plays an essential role in voluntary movement. It is essential to the sustained contraction of skeletal (voluntary) muscles, working at the junction of nerve and muscle. In this action it is opposed, in proper sequence, by dopamine. Theoretically, it can be deduced that the unopposed action of acetylcholine would result in muscle spasm. This may be what happens in myotonia congenita.

The chemical defect in myasthenia gravis is the excessive action of cholinesterase, an enzyme that degrades acetylcholine. Thus, in myasthenia gravis, a person may be able to move or to grasp but, due to excessive action of cholinesterase, he or she may not be able to repeat or sustain such motions as chewing, or to hold a suitcase for more than a few seconds.

Years ago, Jolly observed the similarity between myasthenia gravis and curare poisoning and suggested that the former, like the latter, might be treated with physostigmine, which inhibits cholinesterase. This observation led to the modern treatment of this disorder.[3]

There are other movement disorders that are even less well understood than the ones we have discussed. Among these are muscular dystrophies and atrophies, various kinds of paralyses, and familial diseases of motion. As we learn more about how drugs work, some of these disorders may be treated successfully. More than in any other field, neurotransmitter chemistry will probably lead to dramatic advances in the field of movement disorders.

SUMMARY

For the last three chapters we have dealt with drugs that are concerned with mind and muscle. In the next chapter we shall discuss pain and its relief.

REFERENCES

1 *The Pharmacological Basis of Therapeutics,* (5th ed.), L.S. Goodman and A. Gilman, (eds.), Macmillan, New York. 1975, p. 227.
2 G. C. Cotzias et al., "Aromatic Amino Acids and Modification of Parkinsonism," N. Engl. J. Med.: **276**:374–379 (1967).
3 Goodman and Gilman, op. cit., p. 461.

Chapter 11

Pain Relief in the Elderly

It is ironic that the relief of pain should cause conflict. It seems obvious that pain should be relieved, if quickly by an injection or directly by the taking of a pill, so much the better. Some people seek the relief of pain through self-medication, by some ritual of their own, or by drinking alcohol.

Physicians are in constant conflict with themselves about the appropriateness of pain relief. Too many, in our opinion, settle such inward conflicts by saying in effect, "the patient doesn't have long to live, anyway. He is set in his ways and wants medicine. Why not prescribe for his pain?" Such an attitude is again an example of the "old-age write-off." It may be, in the long run, an example of an old-age "rip-off." Instead of proper examination and explanation, the patient may get a hasty but unwise prescription. It has often occurred this way among patients referred to us. It is true, as pointed out earlier, that many patients, some of them with a dozen unused bottles of medicine, have come to expect nothing but prescriptions. But this expectation is a reflection of the lack of concern of physician and pharmacist and should not be supported mindlessly.

Of course the physician has three duties: (1) to relieve pain, (2) to enhance health, and (3) to prolong life. Often these duties are in conflict. Too often general good health suffers in favor of the other two. For example, we recently saw Mr. W., a basically healthy man with shingles, for a painful neuritis that usually clears spontaneously in a month or so. Though usually active and busy, the patient, with his doctor's support, spent his month vainly seeking relief at the hospital, going to a number of consultants, and taking medicine that did no good. This man was actually made worse by the medical encounter.

It is not at all infrequent that elderly patients are made worse by contact with physician or hospital. Medication, ill-advised laboratory tests, over zealous treatment, invasive procedures, and complicated x-rays all add to the patient's misery and cost. Nowhere is this more true than in prescribing pain medication. Our advice is to use the simplest, least expensive, and least complicated pain relievers as infrequently as possible and in the smallest possible doses.

Any drug can be habit-forming in a person who is disposed to become dependent on drugs. There are people with dependent personalities who are constitutional leaners. They lean on members of their families, they lean on social agencies, on ritual, on alcohol, or on drugs. Some even lean too hard on neighbors or on members of religious groups. Given this overdependence, it is not surprising that people rely too much on drugs, considering the encouragement they are given. We spoke earlier of media advertising of medicine for the relief of nearly every human ailment. Society would be better served, in our opinion, if people were imbued equally with the ideas that every symptom does not reflect disease, that some distress in life is inevitable, and that treatment often does more harm than good.

Among the problems of pain medication are dependency, habituation addiction, and tolerance.

Dependency occurs when a patient becomes dependent on a drug; the drug itself takes on a near-mystical quality, on which some dependent people come to rely. Thus we may find people depending on a "blue heaven" or on a "yellow jacket"—barbiturate medicines nicknamed for the color of their capsules. Long after the medication has lost effectiveness—as many do in a few days—some people still depend on it to promote relaxation or sleep. Many people are dependent on variants of the old APC tablets composed of aspirin, phenacetin, and caffeine. If such medication is discontinued, patients may experience aggravation of symptoms but will not develop acute withdrawal symptoms. They may, however, become rapidly dependent on some other medicine or ritual.

Habituation is like dependency except that habituated people usually seek something more than relief of pain. They may actually seek a state of euphoria or oblivion. Often they are dependent on no single drug but may orchestrate a mixture of drugs seeking to escape life's problems. The habituated person cannot be trusted to take any pain medication or psychoactive drug according to directions. We find ourselves appalled that medications all too often prescribed in extravagant quantities, as if the physician were self-conscious about prescribing half a dozen sleeping capsules. Instead, 50 or 100 capsules are prescribed, more than lethal doses for many sleeping medications, to people who may lose count of how many pills and capsules they have taken.

Then there is the true addict, in whom there is a need and a craving for a drug to maintain a sense of well-being and responsible behavior. Though dependency and habituation occur chiefly in people with personality disorders, true addiction can be induced in almost anyone who takes addicting drugs long enough, usually only a period of several days. Though anyone, even laboratory animals, can become addicted, addiction is more apt to occur in people with preexisting personality disorders. Thus, the addict may share some of the personality traits of the person habituated to or dependent upon drugs.

Drug tolerance occurs when more of a drug is required to produce the same effect a smaller dose once did. In many people dosage will reach a given level and remain the same. For example, we have known people in their eighties who have taken meprobamate in a dose of 400 milligrams four times daily for years. They are addicted in the sense that they would become severely ill if the drug were stopped. As long as such people do not demand new drug experiences, i.e., "highs" in the parlance of the drug culture, it is probably better to continue the drug.

An effective but by no means infallible way to make sure drugs are taken according to direction is to prescribe them in small quantities. Thus if a person is disposed to overmedication he or she is reminded that a dozen pills, say, are supposed to last a dozen days, and that no more will be available any sooner. Perhaps *discipline* is the term that should be applied to both the prescribing and taking of drugs.

Analgesia, insensibility to pain without loss of consciousness, is produced to some extent by analgesics. This group of drugs varies in effect from that of aspirin to that of general anesthetics.

The following classification of pain relievers will be used in this chapter.

I Simple painkillers
   A Drugs with antiinflammatory, antipyretic, and analgesic action
      1 The salicylates
         a Aspirin
         b Sodium salicylate
      2 Salicylate-like
         a Aceteminophen
         b Phenacetin
   B Drugs having principally antiinflammatory action
      1 Phenylbutazone (Butazolidin)
      2 Indomethacin (Indocin)
      3 Ibuprofen (Motrin)
      4 Naproxen (Naprosyn)

  II Drugs useful in the treatment of gout
    A Colchicine
    B Allopurinol
    C Probenecid
 III Narcotic analgesics
    A Morphine and congeners
      1 Morphine
      2 Codeine
      3 Heroin
      4 Dilaudid
      5 Others
    B Meperidine (Demerol) and congeners
    C Methadone and propoxyphene (Darvon)
 IV Sedative Antihistamines
    A Promethazine (Phenergan)
    B Hydroxyzine (Atarax, Vistaril)

Before considering specific drug actions, however, and at the expense of belaboring a point, one should consider a number of human factors. Often we have found that pain is as much a matter of the spirit as of the flesh. All of us, particularly people who are lonely, deprived, and hurting, need human contact and sympathy. Most of us like to talk about what hurts us. Among the most graphic of complainers are physicians, judging by their talk in a locker room or on a parking lot. A physician or nurse with a sprained ankle or an aching ulcer is unlikely to suffer in silence. Yet we tend to be condescending when an old person has pains, which are often aggravated by nagging fears, doubts, and uncertainties. The tendency is to give too little attention and too much medicine.

We have often listened to a recital of symptoms, from headache to constipation to nerves, that seemed to miss the point. Then, when we asked, "Mrs. Jones, what is really upsetting you?" we opened the way to helping. Very possibly, Mrs. Jones had had a death in the family, a slight by a neighbor, or a disappointment by a relative.

These conversations don't take long, on the average, once rapport with a patient is established. They help the physician to prescribe rationally for what may prove to be a short indisposition rather than for a long siege of pain. Understanding and support are often more helpful than medicine. Many physicians feel that they are powerless when confronted with a person with a number of vague aches and pains. In these days of specific treatments for specific illnesses, some physicians—and some patients—are overwhelmed with the need to prescribe or take a number of medicines. When it comes to relieving pain, we have often reminded patients that medicines don't really care what kind of pain they relieve. That is, arthritis medicine may relieve a headache.

The point we wish to emphasize is this: in relieving pain, the attitude and manner of the physician may be more important than the kind or amount of medicine prescribed. We shall have more to say about this aspect of prescribing in another chapter when we talk about placebos.

SIMPLE PAINKILLERS

Salicylates

The salicylates relieve slight to moderate pain, reduce fever, and relieve inflammation.

Aspirin is the best known and probably the most effective, most widely used, and least expensive of the salicylates. It will be used as an example of the whole group.

Aspirin has an action both on the central nervous system and at the site of pain, which is often a locus of inflammation. Irritating and complex chemicals, among them prostaglandins, are produced by the process of inflammation. Aspirin inhibits prostaglandin production. Aspirin also affects pain perception in the lower brain center. This is believed to be so because consciousness, mentation, and sensations other than pain are not disturbed, as when narcotic analgesics are used.

Aspirin is useful to reduce fevers which are of themselves harmful, especially in the very old or the very young. This antipyretic action probably occurs in the temperature-regulating centers of the hypothalamus.

Chronic use of aspirin does not lead to tolerance or addiction. Since it causes no alteration of awareness or sensation, habituation is rare. It has been found in certain circumstances to be as effective, dose for dose, as codeine and Darvon, both of which have a slight tendency to lead to tolerance or addiction. It should be stated, though, that experimental models for the measurement of pain relief are not perfect, especially when one is dealing with chronic, mild to moderate pain.

For most types of common pain, aspirin is apt to be helpful. Most headaches, arthritis, strains and sprains, bumps and bruises, backaches and cricks or catches in the neck are as apt to be relieved by aspirin as by any other reasonable medication. Difficulty arises when patients are intolerant of pain to the point that they prefer oblivion to enduring even a little pain. Only rarely are such patients seen in medical practice. In a geriatrics practice, however, there are usually a few patients who have manipulated physicians into prescribing harmful medicines over a long period of time. Physicians should be wary of going beyond the use of aspirin, or one of its relatives, to relieve chronic pain.

Aspirin is dispensed in many different forms, either alone or in combination with other drugs. One form may give a better result than another for a given patient. Aspirin may be buffered or coated and given in different sizes, shapes, and colors. It is dispensed under at least a dozen different trade names, either alone or in combination with other drugs. For old people who simply need aspirin

(

but who may ache more on a cold, damp day, sometimes a change from one form to another helps, if for no other reason than the placebo effect, which we will discuss in the next chapter.

The most highly advertised painkillers contain aspirin, phenacetin, and caffeine. There is no rationale for such a combination, as time honored as APCs are. Phenacetin has no place in the treatment of disease because of the damage chronic use can do to the kidneys. Caffeine has no pain-relieving qualities.

Aspirin is available in combination with a barbiturate. For a person with temporary restlessness and aching, as with influenza, the combination may be more helpful than aspirin alone. Aspirin is also combined with a number of centrally acting muscle relaxants, mentioned in the last chapter. In our experience, it seems that aspirin alone is about as effective as the far more expensive combination.

It is commonly believed that there is no difference among brands of aspirin. In a purely chemical sense this may be true; i.e., one brand is not superior to another. There is a difference, however, in the hardness of the tablet and the rate at which it disintegrates in the stomach. Certainly, a slowly disintegrating lump of corrosive acid is to be avoided. We have found that the Bayer brand disintegrates rapidly and is better tolerated than some cheaper brands.

Under the best of circumstances, aspirin is irritating to the stomachs of most people. The irritation may be felt as mild nausea or heartburn. In such cases an antacid may relieve the symptoms. In about 70 percent of people who take aspirin regularly, however, there will be some degree of bleeding from the stomach. This bleeding may be inconsequential, but it can be serious if prolonged. It is indeed rare for serious hemorrhage to occur abruptly. Rather, there is more apt to be a slow, persistent loss of blood over a prolonged period of time. An example we recall is of an elderly woman who took a combination medicine containing aspirin for her rheumatism. Over a period of time she became weak, easily fatigued, and pale. A blood count revealed anemia. Only after lengthy observation did it become apparent that her anemia was due to blood loss caused by a disguised form of aspirin. Aspirin should never be given to a person with a bleeding tendency, particularly if that person is taking warfarin (Coumadin), a "blood thinner."

To be fully effective, aspirin should be given in sufficient amount to give a blood plasma level of about 200 micrograms per milliliter. When this level is greatly exceeded, the patient may have an increased loss of blood from the upper gastrointestinal system because of aspirin's irritating effect. Nausea and vomiting may be produced not only because of gastric irritation but also because of aspirin's stimulating effect on the vomit center in the brain.

Among the early symptoms of salicylate intoxication are impaired hearing and tinnitus, an annoying ringing of the ears. It is not unusual for an elderly person with severe arthritis taking 10 or 12 aspirin tablets a day, a total of 3 to 4 grams, to develop ear symptoms. Indeed, if the dose is being pushed, such symptoms can be an early warning sign of intoxication.

In large doses, aspirin can be fatal by its action on the liver, the kidneys, and the central nervous system. Fatal poisoning occurs most often in children, who may confuse colored or flavored aspirin tablets with candy. Aspirin is rarely used in suicide attempts because it inflicts acute suffering before it kills.

In the last few years, aspirin, in small doses, has been used to give a degree of protection against thrombosis. The rationale for such treatment is that to some extent it blocks the tendency of blood platelets to adhere to each other and to the connective tissue fibers of blood vessels. Since aspirin is relatively safe, its use as preventive treatment may be justified. In one case in our experience, however, just two aspirin tablets a day led to harmful bleeding from the stomach and had to be stopped.

Sodium salicylate is almost identical to aspirin in its therapeutic and toxic effects. In spite of the claims of manufacturers, we know of only one advantage: It has a different name and is available in a different form, and may be preferred by a person who insists that aspirin does no good and wants to try something different.

Salicylate-like Drugs

Acetominophen, in our opinion, is the only one of a number of salicylate-like drugs available that should be prescribed. It has a number of dosage forms under a number of trade names, Tylenol being the best-known. Acetominophen equals aspirin in relieving pain that is not accompanied by inflammation. It is useful for headaches and muscular aches. It is used in the same dose as aspirin. The advantages that acetominophen has over aspirin are that it is not as irritating to the stomach and it does not increase the bleeding tendency. On rare occasions, a patient is allergic to aspirin, which may seriously aggravate asthma. Acetominophen, then, would be the drug of choice.

In recent years we have come to believe that acetominophen is the drug of choice for most old people with simple temporary aches and pains. For those who have truly inflamed joints, aspirin remains the mainstay of treatment. There have been a few reports of severe liver damage from massive doses of acetominophen, which indicates it is not a very good poison for suicide. Certainly, it should not be left around for children to eat like candy.

Because of its dangers, we do not believe that *phenacetin* should be used at all.

Antiinflammatory Drugs

We come now to a class of drugs that have principally antiinflammatory action. Such drugs are useful in treating acutely inflamed joints, muscles, and ligaments. They are similar to aspirin in chemical structure.

Phenylbutazone (Butazolidin) was the first such drug to become available on prescription. Although it can, on occasion, give a great deal of relief in painful skeletal disorders, it should be used with caution. Phenylbutazone is irritating to the stomach, depressing to the bone marrow, and dangerous to use in conjunction with warfarin, sulfonamides, and oral hypoglycemic drugs. Its use, unlike aspirin, requires close monitoring even after prolonged use. We have found that when aspirin has failed, phenylbutazone occasionally helps. Indeed, when patients despair and beg to "try something else," then and only then may this drug be used.

Indomethacin is also used in skeletal disorders. Generally, its unpleasant reactions are more frequent but less severe than reactions to phenylbutazone. It causes headache and stomach irritation in a high proportion, perhaps one-third to one-half, of patients who take it. Indomethacin is not clearly superior to aspirin in the treatment of joint disorders but, like other drugs, it is something else to try in discouraged patients.

Both phenylbutazone and indomethacin work by inhibiting the synthesis of prostaglandins at the site of inflammation. From the present state of knowledge it is generally believed that prostaglandins act upon sensitive nerve endings to cause pain in inflammation.

In the last 4 or 5 years a number of other medicines have come on the market, reflecting extensive research in antiinflammatory agents. Among these are *ibuprofen* (Motrin) and *naproxen* (Naprosyn). These drugs are relatively safe, very expensive, and no more effective than aspirin. They do, however, sustain hope in patients who have good reason to become discouraged.

DRUGS USED IN THE TREATMENT OF GOUT

We should state that the antiinflammatory drugs we have mentioned in this chapter thus far may be helpful in gout, which we will now consider in greater detail. Gout is an arthritis-like disease which results from the deposition of irritating uric acid crystals in and around joints and which can be extremely painful. The disease tendency is inherited. Gout is due to one or both of two mechanisms, neither of which is completely understood: (1) excessive uric acid production or (2) insufficient uric acid excretion. The aim of treatment, then, is to rid the body of excess uric acid, to alleviate its effects while still present, and to limit its production.

Colchicine, a classic remedy which dates back at least several hundred years, is used in acute gout. Apparently it reduces the inflammatory response to uric acid deposition. It does not influence uric acid excretion. Colchicine does cause nausea, vomiting, and diarrhea of potentially serious degree, and it should be used only in an acute, severe attack.

Allopurinol, On the other hand, inhibits the production of uric acid. Its use, then, may mobilize uric acid deposits and precipitate an acute attack. Some authorities recommend the concurrent use of colchicine or uricosuric agent (an agent that causes increased excretion of uric acid) during the initial stages of treatment to prevent an acute gouty attack. By the time old patients are referred to us, however, they may have taken gout medicine for years, and we seldom initiate gout treatment.

Probenecid works upon the kidney tubules. It inhibits the reabsorption of uric acid and thus enhances uric acid excretion. (Incidentally, it has an opposite effect on penicillin.) Thus, probenecid may be used with allopurinol.

Neither allopurinol nor probenecid are particularly dangerous. Rarely, both may cause severe skin rashes, stomach distress, or bone marrow depression. For these reasons they require monitoring but they are relatively safe drugs to use.

NARCOTIC ANALGESICS

We have not yet discussed severe visceral pain such as occurs in intestinal obstruction, severe pleurisy, or gallbladder colic. The pain relievers we have mentioned have little effect in such disorders. Usually a narcotic is necessary.

All narcotics have both a legal definition and a number of similar characteristics. They are all habit-forming to some extent as well as addicting, and all have a strong potential for inducing tolerance and euphoria. In sufficient doses, they induce sleep. They are the most potent pain relievers short of general anesthesia. They suppress cough, bowel motility, respiratory and gastrointestinal secretions, and respiration. They are not anticholinergic in a strict sense because their locus of action is, suffice it to say, different. For example, they may constrict pupils and increase tone of bowel musculature. For maximum effect in severe pain they are frequently given along with atropine or promethazine, which have anticholinergic effects.

Morphine and Congeners

Of the narcotics, opium and its derivatives are probably the best known. They work on the central nervous system, but the exact mechanisms are not known. Apparently, they don't work on any well-understood neurotransmitter system. It is interesting that certain opioids, drugs having chemical structures and actions similar to morphine, may be used to counteract morphine overdosage. This suggests some competition with morphine for receptor sites in the central nervous system.

Morphine causes nausea, a fall in blood pressure, and respiratory depression. In our experience, morphine is seldom necessary in old people. Its dangers outweigh its unquestioned effectiveness in relieving pain. We use it promptly, however, when other narcotics fail.

Codeine as a pain reliever is, dose for dose, probably not superior to aspirin except that its reputation for being "strong" may have a psychological benefit to a person in pain. It has the advantage that it can be given by needle. Since it is among the best of cough suppressants, codeine is useful for the aches of influenze, a severe cold, or bronchitis. It is frequently prescribed, alone or in combination with a salicylate, for sprains, headaches, or arthritis. Since it has a potential for addiction, we don't believe it should be used for chronic conditions. The addiction to codeine, to codeine-containing syrups, and to the similar opium derivatives *Percodan* and *Hycodan,* should be suspected when old people ask for renewal of prescriptions of such products. The withdrawal symptoms of these drugs are not to be compared with those of morphine, heroin, or diladid, but they are unpleasant for the patient who has a craving for and a nervous agitation about these medicines.

Heroin is not available legally in the United States. In Great Britain it is said to be more effective than morphine for the terminal care of cancer patients because it produces a greater sense of euphoria and less depression. Of course, euphoria is one reason it is so addictive and is responsible for the commerce in its illegal use.

Paregoric, used principally in relieving diarrhea, is an opium derivative in combination with certain aromatics. It can cause addiction. It is an old drug that is still available, but its use is no longer justified because there are more effective medicines available.

Meperidine and Congeners

Opiates are unsurpassed as pain relievers. Their disadvantages, however, often make other drugs preferable in most situations. *Meperidine* (Demerol) is a widely used synthetic drug which is unlike morphine in chemical sturcture but similar in clinical effect. It is an effective pain reliever, though not as effective as morphine. Its duration of action is shorter. It is not as apt to produce euphoria. Like morphine, it depresses respiration, causes constriction of the pupils, and can cause spasm of gastrointestinal musculature.

Because it is not as depressing to respiration as morphine, Demerol probably is the drug to use first in severe pain of visceral origin in old people. It may cause nausea and vomiting, which tend to subside as pain is relieved. Like morphine, it may be used concurrently with promethazine, which relieves nausea and has pain-relieving properties of its own.

There are other drugs similar in structure and action to Demerol, but we have had no experience with them. They are reported to have no particular advantage.

Methadone and Propoxyphene

Methadone is a synthetic narcotic which was introduced in the late forties. It was at first believed to be an effective pain reliever with few of the disadvantages of morphine and meperidine. Experience soon showed, however, that it had a strong propensity for addiction. It is not used much except in treating heroin addicts, who may experience less euphoria taking methadone than when taking heroin.

Propoxyphene (Darvon) is chemically related to methadone and, roughly speaking, has the same relationship to methadone as codeine bears to morphine. It works on the central nervous system to relieve pain but has no antipyretic or antiinflammatory effect. Like codeine, it has a slight tendency toward addiction. It has no great superiority over aspirin or codeine in our experience. Its chief advantage, as we see it, is that it is another drug useful to instill a measure of hope in discouraged patients. On occasion it may cause dizziness. In compulsive users, propoxyphene may cause a "high" if taken in sufficiently large doses. If withdrawn abruptly after prolonged use, say a month or more, the patient may feel agitated with exaggerated pain. Propoxyphene is at least 15 times as expensive as aspirin and 5 times as expensive as codeine, dose for dose. This difference in cost is seldom justified by the effectiveness of propoxyphene.

Earlier, we spoke of aspirin in combination with salicylate-like drugs. Aspirin augments the pain-reducing properties of codeine and propoxyphene, perhaps by its antiinflammatory action. Six hundred milligrams of aspirin with 65 milligrams of propoxyphene or 600 milligrams of aspirin with 30 milligrams of codeine are apparently more effective than the sum of the individual actions of the components.

SEDATIVE ANTIHISTAMINES

Promethazine

It is not generally appreciated that at least two sedative antihistamines are effective in relieving pain, particularly in old people. Quite often, even in severe pain of unusual origin, *promethazine* gives relief without the nausea, decreased blood pressure, marked stupor, and respiratory depression that are likely from an effective dose of morphine or meperidine. Promethazine is a phenothiazine and is chemically related to a number of antipsychotic drugs. When first introduced in 1946, it was used in allergic conditions such as hay fever. It was then found to have sedative properties and to be effective in controlling the symptoms of motion sickness, chiefly nausea and vomiting. Later, it was used to control nausea in surgical patients. Gradually promethazine has gained limited acceptance as a general purpose drug.

In our view, its virtues are not sufficiently appreciated, particularly in old people. Our practice, and that of others with whom we work, would be much more difficult without promethazine (Phenergan). In small doses, 12.5 milligrams by mouth, it often relieves mild vertigo or nausea. In this dose it can also be used as a mild sedative. Twenty-five milligrams by mouth may cause mild drowsiness but does not cause the euphoria, confusion, and disequilibrium caused by many other sedatives. In acute conditions, including gallbladder disease and acute diverticulitis, it often gives relief without causing nausea or stupor, thus allowing patients to cooperate in the assessment of their pain and general condition.

Promethazine has an anticholinergic action, but not so profound as to cause severe symptoms. An antihistamine, it reduces such histamine effects as dilated blood vessels, gastric hypersecretion, and bronchospasm. Combined with its central nervous system depressing effect, it is an extremely useful drug.

Promethazine may be given in doses up to 50 milligrams intramuscularly or by mouth. This large dose given intramuscularly relieves most severe pain. After a few minutes, say 20 or 30, if a patient has not obtained relief, morphine or meperidine may be given with greater safety than if promethazine had not been given earlier.

To our physician colleagues—and to others—we advise the use of promethazine, a versatile, effective drug for pain and other symptoms in old people.

Hydroxyzine

We have had limited experience with *hydroxyzine*. Though not chemically similar to promethazine, it shares many of its actions. Its effectiveness as a pain-relieving drug probably has been better documented than that of promethazine, although its general usefulness is not so great.

Before leaving a discussion of pain relief in old people, *corticosteroids* should be mentioned. Such drugs are, of course, similar in action to extracts of the adrenal cortex. There are numbers of such drugs, now made synthetically. When they first became available 30 years ago, they were promoted as a boon to arthritis sufferers. Alas, this promise has not been kept. Although they have decided antiinflammatory properties, their side effects can be disastrous. We condemn their use for simple pain relief. They should be used only for serious short-term illness and, on rare occasions, in life-threatening situations.

Now that we have considered pain relief with drugs, we shall devote the next chapter to a discussion of placebos.

Chapter 12

Placebos and Placebo Effects

Webster's Seventh New Collegiate Dictionary defines a placebo as an "inert or innocuous medication given especially to satisfy the patient." An often-overlooked definition is "something tending to soothe or gratify." Too often in the doctor-patient relationship, "soothing" and "gratifying" are excluded in favor of medicines which may not be innocuous.

Prescribing a placebo may be a dirty trick if it is done in a manner that writes off the patient's pain or discomfort, or if it eliminates the opportunity to express pain or anguish. People need to purge themselves of strong feelings—pain, rage, resentment. Old people, nurses, and physicians do not as a rule suffer in silence. Most humans, in appropriate settings, like to talk about themselves.

In a medical setting, people talk about their symptoms. Within limits this is desirable; talk and understanding are therapeutic. If there is doubt of this very human fact, just look at parents and children. In cold scientific terms there is no rationale for hugging and kissing a small child with skinned knees. In human terms, however, the hugging and kissing is "something tending to soothe or gratify." One of the convenience bandage manufacturers speaks of "Band-aids and a little bit of love." The point is that the manner of human interaction is often, but by no means always, as important as the substance.

Some people scorn the use of placebos as being dishonest. Yet serious operations, now discarded as being worthless, were found to be helpful only for their placebo effect. Some patients are so much in need of "doing something" that the placebo effect of having an operation may, on occasion, help out of proportion to any physical benefit. The wise physician or surgeon always tries to separate the placebo effect from true physical benefit in assessing the worth of a procedure or a prescription or an operation. Often, prolonged experience is necessary in making such an assessment.

To some, the prescription of placebos poses an ethical question. Should people pay for inert substances? The answer is that to do so may, on occasion, be the lesser of evils. Should they pay far more for substances, certain tranquilizers for example, which have the potential for making them worse? These questions do not have an easy or categorical answer. Their best resolution depends upon the wisdom of the doctor and the doctor-patient relationship. Certainly, patients and their families have every right to ask what any medicine, placebo or otherwise, is supposed to accomplish and what its pharmacologic action is supposed to be.

If we consider the soothing effects of the power of suggestion, we may learn something about the placebo effect. "I believe the medicine will knock out that pain" uttered by a kindly physician after appropriate questioning and examination of the patient is apt to be effective. The same medicine given without proper attention is apt to have little if any benefit. An elderly patient once told one of us: "That is the best medicine I ever had. I took it home, set it on the dresser and never even took it—and I began to feel better." The point is that he had a chance to talk over his problem and to have it duly respected. He was told that his symptoms were of little consequence and that, if needed, his medicine would help. He had his worry relieved, he was soothed, and the medicine was available if he truly needed it. As it turned out, he didn't.

Why are medicines sold in pretty packages, in tasty-looking colors, and in attractive sizes, shapes, and consistencies? Drug manufacturers know the placebo effect of making medicine look like candy. We have known patients who swore by a bright, attractive medication but got no benefit from the identical substance packaged in a drab, nondescript color. Few people are so coldly scientific that they are not influenced by the sensation of sight, color, form, or consistency. The senses often dictate how we feel or how we look upon our surroundings. The wise physician, therefore, is able to exploit feelings and sensory perceptions to the patient's benefit.

There is an old saying in medicine that a given medicine, including a placebo, will help a third of the patients, will make a third worse, and will have no effect on a third. The idea is to weigh the medicine in favor of benefit by calling upon kindness, sympathy, understanding, and a bit of everyday ritual.

Ritual? Yes! From the most primitive to the most sophisticated of people, humans have their rituals. Medicine men conjuring potions from leaves and roots in the jungle understand that ritual is necessary to have their nostrums work.

Modern physicians need to understand that a sincere and unhurried bedside manner is more effective than a gruff, hurried manner, especially with old people. So the attitude of nurses, physicians, and pharmacists has a great deal to do with whether or not a medicine works.

Placebos should not be given to get rid of a patient. They will not work in such circumstances. If given with love, kindness, and courtesy they will often help. Many old people are convinced that medicine given by injection is more effective than that given by mouth. Old people will remember that sometime, somewhere, they were given an injection that made them feel better. Vitamin B_{12} has long been given for its placebo effect. The disadvantage of B_{12} shots is that they may, on rare occasions, mask serious disease. We have found that an injection of normal saline solution will help some patients who are really asking for an injection of love and understanding. Of course, the injection should be given with love and understanding if it is to help. The effort of another to help is often all discouraged patients need, and if they prefer a harmless injection, why not?

Too often, doctors and nurses are prone to warn, to admonish, or to preach when an old person simply has a need for attention and sympathy. Of course, there are limits to ritual, as to anything else. If, however, placebos make people feel more at peace with themselves and the world, we see no harm in their occasional use.

Like anything else, placebos can be overused. They can cause dependence in susceptible people. Some physicians and nurses deceive themselves into believing that their placebos have true pharmacologic effects. A case in point was the widespread use of procainamide to prevent some of the processes of aging. Another example of placebo effects is the widespread use of certain anticancer drugs which have been shown to have no pharmacologic action.

To the inexperienced it may seem incogruous that we speak of scientific pharmacology and placebos in the same breath, or in the same sentence. Yet it would not only be unscientific but downright stupid to overlook the placebo effect. Indeed, while this book was being prepared, an explanation for the placebo effect was being found. Working something like a conditioned reflex, the expectation of pain relief may cause the brain to secrete pain relieving substances called *endorphins*.

The ultimate test of a drug is made in what is called a *double-blind crossover study*. Such a study takes into account the biases of investigator and subject—biases such as preconceived notions, color and texture, and natural inclinations. Double-blind means that neither subject nor investigator knows whether the subject is taking a potentially active drug or an inert substance, since they are made to appear the same and are distinguishable by a code known only to a third party. So much for double-blind. The crossover means that unknown to subject and investigator, the drug being tested may be substituted for the placebo, or vice versa. Thus the double-blind crossover test is necessary to rule out the placebo effect. It is remarkable how many tests have been made with complex chemicals only to find that they are no more effective than a simple sugar in a pretty colored capsule.

Our contention is that drugs such as Valium and other tranquilizers are often prescribed when only a placebo effect is needed. As great a blessing as antipsychotic drugs are, they are often used for transient episodes of simple nervousness in doses that can do real harm to an old person. Often, tranquilizer pills or sleeping pills are prescribed in such numbers as to be dangerous. We plead for the use of placebos where only placebos are needed.

Less frequently, as in the case of severe emotional disturbance or pain, placebos are prescribed when a more powerful drug is called for. Thus the patient may be given too little or too much. This dilemma can be overcome by closely observing the patient for a period of time before prescribing in quantity.

Rightly used, and with an understanding of the placebo effect, placebos can be helpful in treating many patients. We have used gelbenul (literally, yellow nothing), a yellow capsule, or rotenul (literally, red nothing), a red tablet, with good results for years in patients who only required a placebo. Restraint, reassurance, and appropriate examination are the necessary ingredients of good placebo treatment. Patients fare better than with active but unnecessary treatment.

Chapter 13

Arthritis and Its Treatment

Because various forms of arthritis are so painful and so prevalent, it is appropriate to discuss them at length. The two most troublesome forms of arthritis, as far as prevalence is concerned, are rheumatoid arthritis and osteoarthritis.

In a book like this, it is worthwhile to discuss arthritis treatment because a number of promising drugs have been developed in the last 2 or 3 years. Although it is not clear at present just what role these drugs will play, they should be included for the sake of completeness.

RHEUMATOID ARTHRITIS

Rheumatoid arthritis is a chronic condition which is generally characterized by the symmetric inflammation of peripheral joints. The disease, if progressive, leads to destruction of these joints and their related structures.

The disease, which afflicts about 6½ million Americans, is distributed throughout all age groups. Only 0.2 percent of people under 25 years of age are afflicted by some form of arthritis. Only 10 percent of its victims develop the disease after 50 years of age. By the age of 75, however, there is a 28 percent chance of having some sort of arthritis. The incidence of rheumatoid arthritis and osteoarthritis (which afflicts another 16 million Americans) is increasing because more people are living long enough to develop some form of these disorders.

Rheumatoid arthritis is characterized by morning stiffness, pain and tenderness in the joints, swelling in or about the joints, and subcutaneous nodules of granulomatous tissue with macrophages, necrosis, and fibrosis. A positive agglutination test and osteoporosis are also characteristic. Osteoporosis, the thinning of bone substance, is related to the severity and duration of the disease as well as to the patient's age at the onset. It tends to be more pronounced among the elderly.

Additionally, the condition is influenced by some of the drugs used in treating the disease. Salicylates and corticosteroids, for example, increase bone resorption.

Let us consider some of the effects of the various drugs used to treat rheumatoid arthritis on underlying biochemical markers of the disease, especially prostaglandins, serum acute phase proteins, and hydroxyproline.

Prostaglandins   Synovial tissue, fibrous tissue surrounding joints and tendons, from persons with rheumatoid arthritis produces ten times as much prostaglandin E_2 (PGE_2) as does normal synovial tissue. PGE_2 is a potent inflammatory and osteolytic (bone-destroying) agent, so this diseased tissue tends to destroy underlying bone. Some studies have shown therapeutic serum levels of indomethacin inhibit 90 percent of this excess PGE_2 production. Some of the newer nonsteroidal antiinflammatory agents also possess this action to some degree.

Serum acute phase proteins   The state of rheumatoid arthritis may be assessed by observing changes in levels of serum acute-phase proteins. Patients with severely progressing disease may have consistently higher levels of these proteins than those with mild disease. Improvement or progression may correlate with a fall or rise of these proteins, which may also fluctuate after trauma or inflammation.

One study of the effects of antiinflammatory drugs on acute-phase proteins produced a mixed response. Over a 6-week period, salicylates, indomethacin, phenylbutazone, and ibuprofen had no effect on the erythrocyte sedimentation rate (ESR). The ESR is dependent on the acute-phase protein fibrinogen. They had no effect on the other acute-phase proteins, C-reactive protein, or serum haptoglobin. However, adrenal corticosteroids caused a marked fall of the ESR and the acute-phase proteins. Because the ability to influence measurable substances implies an ability to change the course of the disease, and because nonsteroidal drugs have no effect on these, it seems unlikely that nonsteroidal antiinflammatory agents alter the course of arthritis. This is a basic difference between the two classes of drugs steroidal and nonsteroidal and indicates that they act differently.

Hydroxyproline Collagen is the major protein in connective tissue. Tissue inflammation and repair lead to the production of newly formed and initially soluble collagens, which participate in the body response to, and the repair of, all types of injuries.

Proline is incorporated into the peptide linkage of collagen and is then hydroxylated. Hydroxyproline, which constitutes one-seventh of the amino acid residue of collagen, is very rare in other body proteins. Thus an index of collagen metabolism is the amount of hydroxyproline in body fluids and tissues. There is a direct relationship between the blood and urine content of hydroxyproline and the extent and activity of rheumatic disease. Thus, another measure of antiinflammatory drugs is their inhibiting effect on collagen synthesis in inflammation.

Steroid therapy generally reduces hydroxyproline levels, as do the nonsteroidal antiinflammatory agents phenylbutazone and naproxen. However, with the latter two drugs, there is no change in the erythrocyte sedimentation rate, as pointed out above.

Treatment of Rheumatoid Arthritis

The drugs or drug classes used in rheumatoid arthritis include: (1) gold salts, (2) penicillamine, (3) the antimalarials chloroquine and hydroxychloroquine, (4) steroids, (5) salicylates, and (6) nonsteroidal antiinflammatory drugs other than salicylates, (7) cyclophosphamide.

Gold Gold is generally considered to be most effective in the early and progressive stages of rheumatoid arthritis. In many patients, pain and inflammation are decreased and disability is lessened. X-rays may show the disease to be arrested or improved. Because most of the benefits of gold therapy occur in the active early stages of arthritis, it is not often of any value to older persons. On the other hand, one study found that with large enough doses there is little difference in the proportions of good results seen in the early or the later stages, in which there is more extensive joint destruction.

Adverse reactions to gold increase with the age of the patient and with the duration of the disease. One study found that the average age of patients with toxic symptoms was 47 years and without such symptoms was 41.4. The extent to which toxicity increases with age is not known, probably because gold is not used so often in the elderly. Thus we have a dilemma: gold toxicity increases with age, possibly because slower excretion causes higher blood levels and because older persons require larger doses. Identical doses of gold sodium thiomalate may produce blood levels ranging from 200 to 500 micrograms per 100 milliliters. Individualizing doses to maintain a blood level of 300 micrograms per 100 milliliters produced good results and was well tolerated. Patient ages were not mentioned.

Gold salts should be used very cautiously, if at all, when there is declining cerebral and cardiovascular function, and not at all when there are renal or hepatic disturbances.

Penicillamine   Penicillamine may provide a successful and even superior alternative to gold in the long-term treatment of rheumatoid arthritis, especially in patients who cannot tolerate gold. It has improved the clinical status and the biochemical indices of serum immunoglobulins, ESR, and rheumatoid factor titer and seemingly alters the course of the disease. It also seems to improve bone mineralization so that osteoporosis is reversed in many patients.

Penicillamine must be discontinued in about 25 percent of patients because of hematologic and renal toxicity. Patients receiving penicillamine should have platelet and white blood cell counts every 7 to 14 days for the first few weeks and then at monthly intervals during maintenance therapy. It is probably most effective in younger persons, whose collagen structure is less stable.

Antimalarials—Chloroquine and Hydroxychloroquine   Antimalarials are effective antiinflammatory agents in about one-third of rheumatoid arthritis patients. Improvement is apt to be slow. Three to six months may be needed for maximum benefit. They are most useful in mild early rheumatoid arthritis and are less valuable in older persons with long-standing advanced disease. In chronic use there is danger of retinopathy and blindness. These drugs concentrate in the melanin-containing tissues of the eye, i.e., choroid, retinal pigment, and iris, to a very high degree. Hydroxychloroquine causes less retinal damage than chloroquine, and damage from hydroxychloroquine rarely occurs in the first year. The antimalarials should not be used for more than three months, and opthalmologic studies should be performed before and after therapy.

We have had little experience in prescribing gold, penicillamine, and antimalarial drugs. Occasionally, they have been prescribed previously for patients who come under our care. We can recall no harm being done by stopping these drugs.

Steroids   The use of steroids in patients of any age with rheumatoid arthritis should be limited to those in whom the disease is causing functional incapacity, and then only for the shortest possible time. Steriods were originally derived from the adrenal glands. Later, a number of synthetic drugs were manufactured that varied only slightly in structure from the naturally occurring cortisone. The corticosteroids, as they are called, occasionally cause psychosis or diabetes. They may also cause cardiovascular complications. Cortisone and hydrocortisone cause sodium retention, which may aggravate hypertension, as well as arteriosclerosis, coronary artery disease, and congestive heart failure. The blood pressure has been noted to rise 20 to 40 mmHg, then decline, stabilize, or continue rising in patients on steroids.

Steroids may cause euphoria, an exaggerated sense of well-being, which may be accompanied by increased activity. This may, in turn, be particularly dangerous in patients with coronary arteriosclerosis accompanied by coronary insufficiency. This euphoria can also lead to a psychological dependency. Upon reducing the dose, patients may become irritable, apprehensive, and anxious.

Although patients may complain more about the disease, there is no corresponding physical or biochemical evidence of deterioration.

Steroids are often associated with an increased incidence of osteoporosis, and this, again coupled with increased activity, can lead to compression fractures and other types of broken bones.

Although corticosteroids have been implicated frequently as causing peptic ulcers, this no longer seems to be the case, except when very large doses are used.

There is increased susceptibility to thromboembolic disturbances and to infection during prolonged therapy with steroids. The high prevalence of respiratory infections during this type of therapy necessitates regular checks.

Steroids greatly increase nitrogen excretion, causing a negative nitrogen balance. This is especially likely in patients on poor diets.

One method of reducing the number and severity of steroid side effects without reducing their benefits in chronic therapy is to give either a single daily dose or, preferably, one large dose on alternate days. This alternate-day therapy makes it possible to stop the drug without tapering and without the fatigue, anorexia, and malaise which are apt to occur on stopping daily doses. Dosing every third day is not effective. Alternate-day therapy prevents total suppression of the interacting hypothalamus-pituitary-adrenal system. The steroids dexamethasone and betamethasone have a more prolonged effect than other commonly used steroids and are not recommended for this type of administration.

Although combinations of aspirin and steroids are often used in severe cases of theumatoid arthritis, it should be remembered that corticosteroids increase the rate of salicylate metabolism so that plasma levels of salicylate are lowered.

Salicylates   Aspirin, the most commonly used salicylate, remains the mainstay of drug treatment for rheumatoid arthritis, as about 45 percent of those with it respond satisfactorily. Although many patients have gastrointestinal upsets with aspirin, most are able to tolerate it in one form or another if they continue with it.

The usual dose of aspirin is from 4 to 6 grams a day. To be fully effective, however, the dose should be based on plasma levels and not on a weight or "as needed" basis. Blood levels of 150 micrograms per milliliter are usually required for adequate suppression of the inflammatory reaction. Counting tablets or assessing pain are not as reliable as blood tests in obtaining the best result from treatment.

Older patients cannot always tolerate maximum doses of aspirin. Patients may forget to take a dose or, forgetting, take more than one dose. Occasionally, elderly patients develop deafness or ringing in the ears from too much salicylate. If they continue to take the aspirin, they may faint with rapid heart action, sweating, and low blood pressure. Salicylate poisoning is seldom serious in old people except in true suicide attempts, in which there may be collapse, coma, and death. A much more common problem is the effect of aspirin on the gut lining. On rare occasions there is an acute hemorrhage in the stomach. More often there is an insidious oozing of blood, as pointed out in Chapter 11.

About 70 percent of those taking moderate doses of aspirin will lose about 5 milliliters of blood per day. Another 15 percent lose over 10 milliliters per day. This can lead to an iron-deficiency anemia in those with little iron reserve. All salicylates cause some gastric bleeding. One survey found the following incidences: plain aspirin—65 percent, effervescent aspirin—55 percent sodium salicylate—25 percent, enteric-coated aspirin—32 percent, enteric-coated sodium salicylate—12 percent.

Some consumer advocates claim that all aspirin is alike and that people should buy the cheapest brand. This is poor advice and indicates a degree of ignorance. We must consider how quickly a tablet disintegrates in the stomach. Aspirin particles can cause local erosion and irritation, leading to occult bleeding, especially when tablets slowly disintegrate and remain in the stomach in large chunks. Using low-priced aspirin that leaves lumps of slowly disintegrating acid lying against sensitive mucous membranes can be more costly in the long run than using slightly more expensive higher-quality aspirin. We are favorably impressed by Bayer and Parke-Davis aspirin (used at the Methodist Retirement Home). They seem to engender less distress and fewer complications than cheaper brands we formerly prescribed. This is important in promoting long-term compliance. We must remind ourselves that although anemia resulting from aspirin use is rare, it remains a possibility when people take it repeatedly. There is not a markedly increased incidence of peptic ulcer and little effect on hemoglobin levels when compared to an untreated population. Others have also noted a difference in the acceptability of various brands of aspirin.

Combination Products   Patients should be cautioned to use only plain or buffered aspirin. Combination products with caffeine, phenacetin, or acetaminophen add nothing but cost. Phenacetin and acetaminophen have no effect on the inflammatory reaction. Phenacetin may cause renal problems with prolonged use, as in the treatment of rheumatoid arthritis.

Enteric-coated aspirin is designed to release the drug in the small intestine and thus reduce gastric upset. However, it may be less effective in attaining adequate blood levels. Ecotrin (Smith, Kline, and French's brand of enteric-coated aspirin) produced blood levels similar to or lower than plain aspirin. Enseals (the Lilly brand for enteric-coated aspirin) produced only low or erratic levels. With these differences in results, in products from well-known and reliable companies, the products from lesser-known companies would appear questionable. Since these reports, Lilly has changed its enteric coating to use cellulose acetate phthalate. This material is widely used by the pharmaceutical industry. Lilly feels that the problem of erratic absorption with corresponding erratic blood levels has been corrected. Unfortunately, there are no blood level studies to verify this.

Although the enteric-coated aspirin produces lower blood levels than the same dose of plain aspirin, it should not be disqualified for use if it causes no other problems. What is important is a consistent and predictable response. It is the erratic release of drug that causes problems — a subtherapeutic response without pain relief the first time, followed by toxicity with the next few doses. The number of tablets should be adjusted to give the desired blood level.

Buffered Aspirin   Purists have questioned whether buffered aspirin is any better than plain aspirin in reducing stomach upset. For every such study and advocacy of plain aspirin, we can counter with a number of people who seem to be able to tolerate the buffered product but not the plain aspirin. Whether this is imagination or placebo effect can be debated. But we are dealing with an art as well as a science.

Alkalinization probably protects the stomach mucosa against some damage by forming an ionized salt of aspirin, which cannot penetrate the mucosal cells. Most buffered aspirin formulations (including Bufferin) contain too little antacid to protect the mucosa fully against this erosive process, and so additional antacid should be added. Magnesium and calcium antacids form a poorly soluble and poorly absorbed compound with aspirin and should not be used. Unfortunately, the most common products, Bufferin and Ascriptin and their extra strength versions, use aluminum as well as magnesium antacids in their antacid formulation. Other formulations with soluble antacids present the patient with large doses of sodium.

Choline Magnesium Trisalicylate   (Trilisate) This drug is available only by prescription. Product literature claims that it causes much less fecal blood loss and gastric irritation than aspirin. We have had little experience with it.

Sustained-Release Aspirin   This form of aspirin is no better than plain aspirin in relieving most symptoms. It does offer a few advantages that cause some patients to favor it. It seems to cause less gastric upset and is more convenient to take. It may be taken at 8-hour rather than at 4-hour intervals, a convenience to some people who don't care to carry around medicine. Because of its delayed and prolonged release over the course of a night, it often offers better control of morning stiffness.

Benorylate   This drug is not yet available in the United States. Upon absorption it is hydrolyzed to yield equal weights of aspirin and acetaminophen and so is therapeutically equivalent to aspirin. Although it seems to produce fewer side effects than equivalent doses of aspirin, it is associated with a greater frequency and earlier onset of salicylism when used at the recommended dose of 8 grams a day.

Nonsteroidal Antiinflammatory Drugs

Indomethacin   This drug is a potent inhibitor of prostaglandin synthetase. In younger persons with rheumatoid arthritis, it produces striking improvement in about 25 percent and worthwhile improvement in another 25 percent. But it is fully effective in only a small proportion of aged arthritics. There is a higher incidence of side effects in the elderly, especially in those over 70 years of age. These major side effects affect the central nervous system with headaches, dizziness, and giddiness and the gastrointestinal system with nausea, vomiting, and peptic ulcers. Peptic ulcers appear in about 3 percent of patients who take indomethacin regularly, and are a contraindication to further use of the drug. Skin rashes may occur, and vasculitis, hypertension, and coronary occlusion have been reported as untoward reactions. Salt retention may occur although edema is rare. Even minimal doses may cause headaches and dyspnea. Because of its potential for adverse effects, indomethacin should not be used indiscriminately or routinely. It should be used for trial periods in patients who either do not respond to rest, physical therapy, or other nonsteroidal antiinflammatory drugs, or who have flare-ups of disease but are otherwise well controlled.

Indomethacin is sometimes used with aspirin. There is some disagreement over the effects of aspirin on indomethacin. One study found that aspirin reduced indomethacin blood levels but others found no such effects.

Morning stiffness is a sensitive indicator of drug efficacy in rheumatoid arthritis. A combination of indomethacin and diazepam may enhance sleep and reduce the pain and duration of morning stiffness. In contrast, diazepam alone, given at night, actually increases morning stiffness.

Phenylbutazone and Oxyphenbutazone   These are of relatively little value in the aged person with rheumatoid arthritis. Symptomatic relief is often poor or of short duration. As with indomethacin, they should be reserved for short-term use in acute flare-ups of the disease when other therapy is inadequate. Their use for more than 5 days is rarely warranted, and they should not be used for long-term pain relief.

The actual incidence of side effects and toxicity, which seem to increase greatly after the age of 40, is less than with indomethacin. Because the minor side effects are less frequent, phenylbutazone is often preferred by many patients. There are, however, a number of serious side effects. None of the other nonsteroidal antiinflammatory drugs can compare with these two drugs in the variety and severity of untoward reactions. There is a fairly high incidence of gastrointestinal, hematologic, fluid and electrolyte, central nervous system, cardiovascular, allergic, and dermatologic complications. An acid-stimulating effect can lead to peptic ulcers and their complications, i.e., perforation and hemorrhage. Retention of sodium and water causes edema and is a definite indication to stop the drug. Central nervous system effects include agitation, lethargy, confusion, depression, psychosis, and insomnia, all of which may be misinterpreted as being due to a failing brain. This may lead to more, not less, treatment with drugs. Patients should be kept under close medical supervision.

Until the past few years the only nonsteroidal antiinflammatory drugs for the symptomatic relief of the various forms of arthritis were the previously discussed aspirin, indomethacin, phenylbutazone, and oxyphenbutazone. While aspirin is usually safe, cheap, and effective, it has a high incidence of gastrointestinal side

effects. Indomethacin, phenylbutazone, and oxyphenbutazone have a high incidence of side effects, and those that occur may be far more serious. Thus, they
have only limited use in elderly patients. In addition, they are much more
expensive than salicylates.

These drugs are now joined by a variety of acetic and propionic acid derivatives. They approximate aspirin in efficacy at maximum therapeutic doses, have
fewer side effects, and cost much more. Because aspirin is the standard drug,
these newer agents are generally compared with aspirin and, to a lesser extent,
with each other. The determination of the efficacy of these drugs involves measurements of pain relief, duration of morning stiffness, onset of afternoon
fatigue, number of swollen joints, grip strength, walking time, and subjective
evaluation by the patients of their overall well-being.

The cost difference of the drugs within this category is considerable. The
daily cost of aspirin is a few cents. That of the larger doses of the newer agents
may be over a dollar a day.

A number of studies have been performed showing a certain daily dose of
one drug to be superior to a certain daily dose of another drug. Not surprisingly, a
maximum dose of one drug is often more effective than a minimum dose of
another. The reader should be aware of the recommended dose ranges shown in
Table 13-1.

All of these drugs induce three major groups of adverse effects with the
major differences being in the incidence and severity of these effects. *Gastrointestinal* effects include nausea, vomiting, cramps, abdominal pain, constipation,
diarrhea, occult blood loss, and activation or exacerbation of peptic ulcers.
Central nervous system effects include dizziness, headache, nervousness, depression, anorexia, somnolence, tremors, and confusion. *Dermatologic* problems include pruritis, rash, hives, urticaria, oral ulcers, and sweating. The incidence and severity of these effects are often dose-related.

Fenoprofen   Fenoprofen may be marginally superior to aspirin in some
ways and inferior in others. It may provide superior pain relief; but when daily
doses of 2.1 grams of fenoprofen were compared with 4.5 grams of aspirin,
aspirin was found to be superior in relieving the duration and severity of morning
stiffness and in improving walking time and grip strength. Aspirin also caused
twice as many side effects. Combined treatment with 3.0 grams of fenoprofen
and 6 grams of aspirin resulted in superior improvement than when aspirin was
used alone. Other studies found that fenoprofen was preferred by 70 percent of
the patients when compared with aspirin.

Side effects of fenoprofen which may be overlooked or attributed to an older
person's age include nervousness, fatigue, dizziness, confusion, malaise,
dysuria, headaches, insomnia, and, in about 4 percent, palpitations and
tachycardia. When administered with aspirin, peak serum levels are reduced
because of aspirin-induced enzyme induction.

Ibuprofen   Ibuprofen was the first of these newer drugs to be used in the
United States. The dose is an important determinant of its efficacy. While some
investigators find that 600 to 900 milligrams per day is not better than a placebo,

others find that 600 milligrams per day is an effective daily dose. Daily doses of 1200 milligrams are primarily analgesic, and about 1800 milligrams per day are required for an antiinflammatory effect. Daily doses of 1600 milligrams per day are only slightly more effective than 3.6 grams of aspirin.

In osteoarthritis, 1200 milligrams of ibuprofen per day is slightly inferior to 75 milligrams of indomethacin, but it causes fewer side effects. In a 6-month double-blind study in 232 patients, 75 to 150 milligrams of indomethacin and 900 to 1800 milligrams of ibuprofen were prescribed. Fourteen patients on indomethacin and four on ibuprofen stopped treatment because of unpleasant side effects. Another study comparing the drugs in rheumatoid arthritis found patients and investigators agreeing that there was no difference in the efficacy of the drugs. However, ibuprofen caused only about 60 percent as many side effects as indomethacin. A dose of 1200 milligrams per day of ibuprofen was not statistically different from 600 milligrams of phenylbutazone per day in relieving pain of movement, spontaneous pain, and morning stiffness, and in improving grip strength and function.

Naproxen   This drug is useful both for long-term management and acute flare-ups of rheumatoid arthritis, as well as for osteoarthritis and ankylosing spondylitis. Naproxen is fully absorbed from the gastrointestinal tract. As the dose is increased the blood level rises linearly up to a maximum dose of 500 milligrams. Initially, only about 0.4 percent of the drug is not bound to plasma proteins. About this dose of 500 milligrams per day, the plasma-binding sites are saturated, and so the unbound proportion of drug rises. This unbound fraction is quickly metabolized and excreted so that doses over 500 milligrams per day result in little change in blood level or therapeutic response. Doses of over a gram a day are wasted. Food will delay drug absorption slightly, but peak plasma levels and the total amount absorbed are not significantly different.

Antacids have a variable effect on the absorption of naproxen. Sodium bicarbonate increases the rate of absorption. Magnesium carbonate reduces absorption slightly. Magnesium oxide and aluminum hydroxide reduce the rate of absorption but not the extent. The peak serum level is lower, but the duration of action is longer. Doses of 400 to 750 milligrams may allow a reduction in the dose of oral corticosteroids in some patients. The greatest potential for drug interactions arises from the competition for transport sites between naproxen and other drugs bound to albumin.

It has been postulated that naproxen may lead to a loss of diabetic control in patients on sulfonylureas and to hypoprothrombinemia in those on warfarin. Administration of naproxen with phenytoin may lead to phenytoin toxicity. Administration of aspirin with naproxen lowers the serum level of the latter. This occurs since aspirin displaces naproxen from serum binding sites so that the latter is metabolized and excreted faster. Clinical trials, however, demonstrate that these drugs have an additive effect.

Gastrointestinal side effects occur in about 14 percent of patients on naproxen. In addition to the general side effects of all of these drugs, naproxen may cause stomatitis, melena, and degeneration of gastric mucosa. The incidence of gastric side effects is less than with aspirin. Gastroscopic comparisons found 12 cases of some degree of gastric pathology in 12 healthy volunteers taking 4.8 grams of aspirin daily. Only 1 in 12 of those taking 500 milligrams of naproxen daily had positive gastroscopic findings. Gastric erosion occurs whether naproxen is given orally or by injection, indicating that it exerts systemic as well as local or topical effects, as do indomethacin and phenylbutazone. Substituting naproxen for aspirin in gastrointestinal bleeding results in a rapid and statistically significant reduction in microscopic bleeding to nearly normal levels. There is no correlation between prolongation of bleeding time and plasma levels of aspirin or naproxen. However, both drugs prolong bleeding time. In the central nervous system, as with related drugs, naproxen can cause lightheadedness and drowsiness. There are also occasional reports of depression and hearing disturbances, which occur in about 8 percent. Dermatologic effects occur in about 5 percent. There are cardiovascular problems in about 2 percent. They include edema, palpitations, and dyspnea.

The contraindications to the use of naproxen are the same as for aspirin. The drug should be used under close supervision, if at all, in patients with gastrointestinal bleeding or disease, in those on coumarin anticoagulants, hydantoin derivatives, sulfonamides, or sulfonylureas, or in those with renal impairment.

There is little therapeutic difference between aspirin and naproxen when comparing overall efficacy or individual criteria of grip strength, pain, or morning stiffness. Naproxen, however, has significantly fewer side effects, and fewer people discontinue treatment with naproxen than with aspirin. Naproxen and indomethacin are also about equal in relief of the symptoms of rheumatoid arthritis and osteoarthritis. They provide the same degree of pain relief and improved range of motion in a variety of tests. As an inhibitor of prostaglandin synthesis, naproxen ranks between indomethacin and aspirin.

Tolmetin Tolmetin is also indicated in the long-term management and flare-ups of rheumatoid arthritis. Dosing intervals are every 8 hours. There is no advantage in shorter dosing periods. Therapeutic response usually appears in about 3 days, but steady improvement may occur over as long as 9 months. Gastrointestinal side effects occur in about one-third of the patients and cause about 10 percent to discontinue the drug. The other major side effects are headaches, tenseness, nervousness, drowsiness, and vertigo.

Patient Compliance Patient compliance with therapeutic regimens for these drugs can be considered from the following aspects: (1) the incidence and severity of adverse effects; (2) the frequency of doses; and (3) the cost, availability, and convenience.

The salicylates are inexpensive and readily available without prescription. They have a high incidence of GI upset, and effective therapy may require up to 15 tablets a day spread over 4 to 5 doses. Extended-release tablets are both more convenient and more expensive. Benorylate, a liquid, may be inconvenient to carry for an active person, and there is a greater frequency and an earlier onset of salicylism. The incidence of side effects is not less than with aspirin.

One product offering convenience of dosage is naproxen, which needs to be taken only twice a day. The adverse effects of indomethacin and, in particular, phenylbutazone are often more serious than with other drugs, and they may force the patient to stop medication. It is difficult to compare the incidence of adverse effects and their severity among the newer agents because the incidence varies among different studies and at different doses. Although the adverse effects may be uncomfortable, they are not usually serious or life-threatening.

Cost Considerations   A final and possibly decisive factor in selecting the drug therapy is cost. Because many arthritics are older, retired, and on a fixed income, they may not be able to afford the more expensive drugs. This is especially true in chronic diseases. Patients may find that they cannot afford the medicine, or they may take it in suboptimal quantities, leading to therapeutic failure. We have heard of patients who go without adequate food in order to purchase medication. The physician and pharmacist should work with the patient to keep drug prices down so that the patient is not deprived of other essentials of life.

Table 13-1 gives average wholesale costs per 100 tablets of various nonsteroidal antiinflammatory drugs and a range of daily costs. The price to the patient will be higher, depending on the pharmacist's margin of profit.

OSTEOARTHRITIS

Osteoarthritis is characterized by the degeneration and loss of joint cartilage, spreading of bone and cartilage at joint edges, and inflammation and pain in joints. The incidence of the disease increases with age, and by the age of 60, about 60 percent of the U.S. population have characteristic pathological, chemical, and radiological changes of osteoarthritis.

The various treatments for osteoarthritis include rest, heat, exercise, weight loss, and drugs. The drugs used to treat the symptoms of osteoarthritis include many of those used in treating rheumatoid arthritis. In particular, these are salicylates, indomethacin, phenylbutazone, and other nonsteroidal antiinflammatory agents. The symptoms of the disease are due to primary degenerative changes and to the secondary inflammation. The chief need is for pain relief.

Oral steroids are not believed to have a role in the treatment of osteoarthritis despite the fact that they provide good pain relief and suppression of inflammation. Their side effects contraindicate their use. Intraarticular injection of steroids may give pain relief for days to months but with no change in the progress of the disease. Intraarticular injection of steroids tends to destroy the remaining articular cartilage by inhibiting matrix synthesis. Large, deformed, relatively painless and useless joints may result. Such joints are called Charcot joints for the French physician who first described them.

Table 13-1 Wholesale Cost of Nonsteroidal Antiinflammatory Drugs

Drug	Trade name and source	Strength, mg	Cost per 100, $	Daily dosage, mg	Wholesale Daily cost, cents
Aspirin	Various	325	—	3000–5000	5–10
Indomethacin	Indocin (MSD)	25	11.80	75–150	35–60
		50	18.83		
Phenylbutazone	Butazolidin (Geigy)	100	9.35	300	28
Ibuprofen	Motrin (Upjohn)	300	10.70	900–2400	33–80
		400	13.00		
Fenoprofen	Nalfon (Djsta)	300	8.60	2400	70
Naproxen	Naprosyn (Syntex)	250	20.20	500–750	40–60
Tolmetin	Tolectin (McNeil)	200	11.90	600–1800	36–107

Chapter 14

Infections in the Elderly

It is not our purpose here to have a general discussion of the treatment of infections. Moreover, with changing patterns of bacterial sensitivity and resistance, and the regular appearance of new antibiotics from research laboratories, such a discussion would soon be out of date.

PRINCIPLES OF TREATMENT

The principles of treatment of infections in old people are basically the same as in the young. The task is, when possible, to identify the infecting agent and to prescribe the most effective treatment. There are, however, a number of problems peculiar to elderly people who may become infected. Some of these are: (1) nutritional state, (2) immunologic status, (3) the presence of other disease, (4) deteriorating physiologic mechanisms, and (5) mechanisms which may predispose to adverse drug reaction. All of these influence and are influenced by infections and their treatment. Figure 14-1 may be useful in understanding interdependent influences in an infected old person.

Nutritional State

The nutritional state may determine how well the body can combat an infection. People with protein deficiencies are unable to make adequate amounts of circulat-

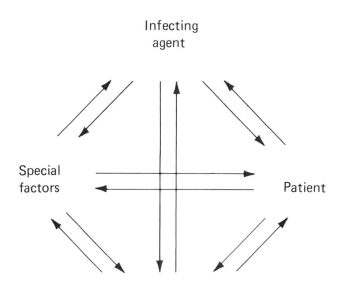

Infecting
agent

Special
factors

Patient

Treatment

Figure 14-1 Interrelated influences in infection.

ing antibodies which neutralize infecting agents, bacteria, viruses, and fungi. Deficiencies of A, B, and C vitamins tend to depress antibody formation. In addition to circulating antibodies, cell–mediated immunity and phagocytic activity are also reduced in the malnourished patient. In a malnourished patient, an infection is apt to be more severe and to last longer than in a well-nourished patient.

The problem is compounded because an infection makes it difficult or impossible for a patient to consume and assimilate a good diet. Ironically, certain parasites are reluctant to establish habitation in a protein-deficient patient. It is as if they were epicures, choosing only the best for their menus. However, in general, malnourished people are far more apt to be the victims of infectious agents.

Deficiencies of vitamins A, B, and C do affect resistance, although the exact mechanisms are not known. Apparently the vitamins don't have a direct influence on antibody production. They may work by their essential roles in the metabolism of other foodstuffs, which does affect the production of cellular and circulating antibodies.

The incidence of malnutrition among the old is not precisely known. When one sees the dry skin, slick tongues, diarrhea, neuritis, mental confusion, and easy bruisability of many old patients, one cannot escape the conclusion that malnutrition is fairly common. Though poverty is a factor, it is seldom the reason for suboptimal nutrition. The chief reason seems to be simply that many old people just don't get hungry. When they do eat, they may choose something they like or something which is easy to fix, such as milk and cereal or canned apple sauce. Loneliness, in which a person has no social reason to eat, may be a factor in malnutrition. Then, too, a person may be unable to chew or to digest adequately because of absent or ill-fitting teeth or too little acid in the stomach. One of the more frequent causes of malnutrition is the fact that many people take medicines which affect nutrition. Many medicines, particularly digitalis, potassium, sedatives, and anticholinergics, take away the appetite or dull the sensorium to the point that a person simply can't or won't eat. Iron tablets often irritate the stomach. Dioctyl sodium sulfosuccinate, a stool softener, depresses stomach secretion. Mineral oil may reduce absorption of important vitamins and minerals.

Nutrition and health are related to each other but also to age, income, education, and residence. Often, the deficiencies become obvious only in institutions such as nursing homes and hospitals.

Immunologic Status

Even with an optimum diet, immunity tends to decline with age, and resistance to infection weakens. Let's talk about the immune system briefly. It is composed of three components: (1) a cellular process, (2) a humoral process, and (3) a phagocytic process.

The *cellular process* concerns itself with delayed reactions. It is mediated by *T lymphocytes*, or T cells, which have been produced or altered by the thymus gland. It is these T cells which are responsible for delayed allergic reaction to certain antigens, and protection against cancer cells and certain fungi, viruses, and bacteria. These T cell immune responses are much less pronounced in people over 60 than in those under 20.

The *humoral process* is mediated by *B lymphocytes*, which are derived from bone marrow stem cells. The B cells produce circulating antibodies, i.e., immune globulins with a high degree of specificity for a particular antigen. This process, as inexorably as others, declines with age.

One theory of aging, among several, is that aging itself is the result of immunologic decline, which predisposes a person to more degenerative diseases and more severe infections.

The *phagocytic process* is simply a process by which one cell surrounds and destroys another. A white blood cell may surround a bacterial cell and, by chemical interaction, dissolve (lyse) it. The vigor of phagocytosis may diminish with age or with diabetes, alcoholism, malignancy, or the use of certain drugs.

Presence of Other Disease

Certainly, concurrent disease influences the response of an old person to an infection. Arteriosclerotic cardiovascular disease frequently predisposes to infection and complicates its treatment. Sluggish circulation may decrease resistance to infectious organisms at a portal of entry, e.g., lungs, skin, or reduce the transport of a blood-borne antibiotic to an infected site. The large amounts of sodium and potassium in many antibiotics may aggravate heart, lung, or kidney conditions.

Compared to arthritis in its several forms, severe infections are in general, rare. However, a number of rare infections are relatively common in old people. Tuberculosis is, nowadays, a rarity except in old people, who may be immunologically compromised, as mentioned above. Periodic chest x-rays in old people are desirable and are required by law in some states for those living in institutions.

Deteriorating Physiologic Mechanisms

Many extremely feeble old people are at risk from aspiration pneumonia because of weakness of the swallowing and coughing mechanisms. This kind of infection, resulting from simple "choking," is far more prevalent than is generally appreciated. Pneumonias of several types, purulent meningitis, and urinary tract infections are more prevalent and more severe in old people.

SPECIFIC DISEASE

Now we wish to discuss particular infections in greater detail, beginning with meningitis.

Meningitis

The meninges are the membranes that protect the brain and spinal cord. Thus we have the ancient, incomplete term "spinal meningitis," which has been adopted as a synonym for meningococcal meningitis, by far the most frequent type in the population as a whole. The greater incidence of chronic disease in the old, combined with their circulatory and immunologic impairments, predisposes them to a relatively high incidence of meningitis from organisms of relatively low virulence, such as *Klebsiella, Proteus,* and *Pseudomonas,* which may be found normally on the skin or in the lower digestive tract. Pneumococcal meningitis, caused by the same organism that causes about 90 percent of pneumonias, is also relatively frequent.

Tuberculosis

Tuberculosis is rarely seen these days except in old people. The reasons for this are the long time between exposure to the organism and the development of the disease. In some cases there can be nearly a lifetime between exposure and disease. The infection may be dormant for years only to become obvious, i.e., symptomatic, when a person is enfeebled immunologically. Another reason for a relatively high incidence of tuberculosis among the old is the reinfection phenomenon. In the days when old people were growing up, nearly 95 percent, at some time, were exposed to tuberculosis, i.e., became infected, mostly unknown to themselves or others. Only after months or years were they reinfected to develop the disease. Due to this bit of natural history of the disease, old people are much more vulnerable than younger people, most of whom never recieved a primary infection. Of course, chronic illness, malnutrition, and alcoholism predispose to the activation of a long-dormant tuberculosis infection.

Modern treatment of tuberculosis prevents the long hospitalization, prolonged illness, and premature death that were formally the hallmarks of the disease. Isoniazid (isonicotinic hydrazide, INH) is the mainstay of treatment. INH is acetylated at varying rates in the liver. Slow acetylators obviously tend to have higher blood levels of the unconjugated drug for longer times and, therefore, are more subject to toxicity than fast acetylators. This toxicity in slow acetylators is manifested as a painful and potentially disabling neuritis. In addition, INH can induce a pyridoxine-deficiency anemia. (Pyridoxine is one of the B vitamins.)

In contrast to the slow acetylators, fast acetylators are more prone to develop liver disease from INH. This hepatotoxicity seems to be related to age, being on the order of 2.3 percent in people over 50 but extremely rare in adolescents. The routine prophylactic use of INH in people over 35 is not recommended. In those at high risk, however, the possible benefit may outweigh the danger. People whose TB skin test has recently changed from negative to positive are considered to be high-risk patients if they undergo treatment with cortisone or other drugs that depress immune response. Other high-risk factors are diabetes, leukemia, Hodgkin's disease, or close contact with a person who has tuberculosis.

Other drugs are used in the treatment of tuberculosis, but we have had little experience with them. Their use is largely restricted to physicians having special knowledge. Among these drugs are ethambutol, cycloserine, viomycin, streptomycin, pyrazinamide, para-aminosalicylic acid (PAS), ethionamide, capreomycin, kanamycin, and rifampin.

Septicemia

Old people are more prone than young people to develop blood stream infections, i.e., bacteremia, and serious illness from such infections, i.e., septicemia. Among the bacteria causing septicemia are gram-negative (pink-staining using Gram's stain) bacilli and such gram-positive (purple-staining using Gram's stain) organisms as staphylococci, streptococci, and pneumococci. The mortality in treated cases of septicemia is appallingly high, ranging from 26 to 80 percent, depending on the organism. The mortality rate rises rapidly after the age of 40. Instead of the chills, fever, and prostration usually seen in severe infections, old people may simply become confused, delirious, agitated, or stuporous, but without fever.

The old person may become dehydrated and fail to excrete urine. The thirst and appetite may diminish. Indeed, the nurse may report that ''the patient is just not acting right today.'' A physician hearing such a report should be aware of the possiblity of a serious infection.

One serious complication of gram-negative septicemia is endotoxic shock. This is a clinical state largely confined to old people. According to theory and to animal experiments, it is due to the release of toxic substances (endotoxins) from the walls of gram-negative bacilli, usually colon bacilli. Clinically, the patient, nearly always of advanced age, is weak, delirious, and hypotensive. The shock state has a very high mortality. Interestingly, it is due to organisms that in their normal habitat do little or no harm. The overuse of certain antibiotics, including penicillin, may have increased the incidence of certain severe infections because of the emergence of resistant strains of bacteria.

Pneumonia

Pneumonia is far more frequent and more serious in old people. The mortality rate is certainly higher, and, when recovery occurs, it is apt to be slower than in younger people. If a person past 65 develops a deep chest cough, sharp pain in the chest, purulent sputum, prostration, fever, or some combination of these symptoms, it may be prudent not to insist on diagnostic precision before starting a broad-spectrum antibiotic. We usually start giving ampicillin before blood and sputum are collected for study. Any patient who gets worse, or is not better in a day or two, is promptly hospitalized.

If the above symptoms develop during the course of an influenza epidemic they should be treated with extreme seriousness. Influenza rarely kills anyone but old people. We vividly remember the Asian flu epidemic of 1969, in which many elderly people died in spite of immunization. It has been shown repeatedly that flu vaccine is about 70 to 75 percent effective in preventing flu and its complications. This is why we recommend its use in old people, particularly in those who live in proximity to each other, as in nursing homes, hospitals, and retirement communities. It is unfortunate that the Hong Kong flu immunization debacle of 1976 tended to discredit all flu immunization.

The geriatric patient is more susceptible to complications of pneumonia for a number of reasons discussed earlier. In addition, there is a general reduction of pulmonary function in old age. Coughing reflexes and the physical strength needed to raise sputum may be reduced. The mucus and cilia that tend to rid the bronchial tubes of foreign matter may not function as well in old age. There may be preexisting lung disease such as chronic bronchitis, asthma, and bronchiectasis. Circulatory disorders such as heart disease or pulmonary emboli make the pneumonia patient even more vulnerable. Complications of pneumonia are much more frequent in old people. These include lung abscesses, meningitis, septicemia with distant abscesses, and others.

The clinical features of pneumonia may vary according to the infecting organism, though in most cases it is unreliable to make an etiologic diagnosis on the basis of clinical findings. It is far better to get some sputum, blood, or both to culture for microorganisms. Then, with a precise diagnosis, treatment can be directed more intelligently.

Up to 90 percent of pneumonias diagnosed by chest x-rays are caused by *Diplococcus pneumoniae*. A few such organisms are normal inhabitants of the respiratory system. When, for reasons not entirely understood, resistance is lowered, or when the organisms become unusually virulent and multiply rapidly, pneumococci, as they are called, can cause serious or even fatal pneumonia.

Mycoplasma pneumoniae is a special breed of organism that causes flulike symptoms. Indeed, infection with *Mycoplasma pneumoniae* should be suspected when flulike symptoms persist for more than a week.

Hospital-acquired Infections

In recent years it has become evident that hospitals are risky places for people, particularly old people. Hospitals are reservoirs of a number of microorganisms that seldom infect people outside hospitals. Among these organisms are certain strains of staphylococci and a number of gram-negative bacilli such as *Pseudomonas* and *Klebsiella*. These hospital infections are frequently airborne or waterborne and may be transmitted, in spite of precautions, by suctioning, intubating, catheterizing, administering fluids, and giving oxygen. Old people are particularly susceptible to such infections for a variety of reasons, as discussed above.

While naturally occurring extrahospital infections have a low mortality, generally 2 or 3 percent, severe infections contracted in the hospital may have a mortality of up to 50 percent. Most adults have heard of a healthy old person going to the hospital for an accident, say, and dying in a week of pneumonia. Except where essential to treatment for particular illnesses, people should avoid hospitals.

Urinary Tract Infections

Urinary tract infections are much more severe and much more frequent in old people. Many infections of the bladder or the prostate are merely troublesome and stubborn annoyances to otherwise healthy old people. However, such relatively innocuous infections frequently became abruptly worse with high fevers and prostration, and for no apparent reason.

Among the reasons for urinary infections in old people are fallen bladders in women and prostate-gland enlargement in men. In addition, urine flow may be reduced. People tend not to drink enough fluid as they get older. The urine acidity tends to fall in old age, favoring bacterial growth. In one study among patients in a nursing home, women had a 27 percent and men had a 17 percent incidence of urinary tract infection. Among the old, it is wise not to treat infections that cause little or no trouble. To do so encourages the emergence of resistant strains of bacteria, which may be dangerous. Treatment, generally, is directed toward relieving symptoms, correcting obstruction (as from an enlarged prostate), giving acidifying agents such as mandelic acid, and encouraging fluid intake.

The most frequent urinary infections are caused by *E. coli, Proteus, Klebsiella,* and *Pseudomonas,* all of which are usually normal flora in the colon. They may develop virulent strains or the aged host may have reduced resistance to them. Only 20 to 30 percent of such infections are cured outright by antibiotic treatment; the remainder develop resistance, or new strains of bacteria emerge. The proper treatment is to follow the general measures above and to use antibiotics only for short periods when the symptoms, e.g., high fever, are truly serious.

Since resistant strains of bacteria are not apt to develop during their use, such sulfonamide drugs as Gantrisin, Bactrim, or Septra may be used prophylactically. Nitrofurantoin is useful in many short-term infections.

Many people have urinary infections which are confined to the bladder. Although troublesome, such infections are usually not considered serious. They require only simple treatment such as a sulfonamide. The danger in such infections is that they will spread to the kidneys. When such spreading occurs, the infection is potentially serious and might require urine culture and sensitivity tests to indicate the probable response to one or several antibiotics.

We shall now discuss a number of antibiotics used in urinary tract infections.

Aminoglycosides This class of drugs includes amikacin, gentamicin, kanamycin, neomycin, tobramycin, and streptomycin. These drugs are generally effective against *Proteus, Enterobacter,* and Klebsiella. Gentamicin and tobramycin are also effective against *Pseudomonas.* They are all nephrotoxic and ototoxic; that is, they can damage the kidneys and the ears. We vividly recall Mrs. X., a patient in her late 70's, who developed appendicitis. In the course of treatment, she was given a gentamicin. She developed uremia, moderate deafness, and constant vertigo. The last two effects are permanent, disabling, and have no known treatment. We wonder if the gentamicin treatment was really necessary. We have been struck by the frequency of use of this drug; whose dangers are not fully appreciated.

Ampicillin Ampicillin achieves effective drug levels in the urine. It is effective against most penicillin-senstive organisms and against *E. coli* and *Proteus mirabilis.* However, it is ineffective against *Enterobacter, Pseudomonas,* and *Klebsiella.* Its side effects commonly include skin rashes and rarely include serious allergic reactions.

Carbenicillin Carbenicillin is effective against *Pseudomonas* and *Proteus* and, unlike other antibiotics effective against these organisms, is not nephrotoxic. Unfortunately, resistance develops rapidly.

Cephalosporins These include cephalexin, cephaloridine, cephaloglycin, cephalothin, cefazolin, cephradine, against *Pseudomonas*, *Enterobacter*, *Serratia*, *Proteus*, and a few others. *E. coli*, which is usually susceptible to cephalosporins, may develop resistance by elaborating cephalosporinase. These drugs exhibit some renal toxicity and must be used cautiously in patients with decreased renal function, or when other nephrotoxic drugs, such as the aminoglycosides, are also used. The use of these drugs along with such potent diuretics as ethacrynic acid or furosemide also increases the possibility of nephrotoxicity.

Methenamine Salts These include methenamine mandelate and methenamine hippurate. Methenamine is broken down to formaldehyde in an acid urine, and it is this formaldehyde which exerts an antibacterial effect. The second half of the salt, the mandelate or hippurate, supposedly provides the acidity necessary to do this. It is often necessary to administer an acidifying agent, such as ascorbic acid.

Nalidixic Acid This drug is effective against most coliform bacteria. A notable exception is *Pseudomonas*. Its use is limited by the rapid development of resistance. It is primarily excreted by the kidneys, but full doses have been used without toxicity in some cases of severe renal failure. Toxic psychosis or convulsions have rarely occurred, usually with excessive doses or in the presence of cerebral arteriosclerosis.

Nitrofurantoin Except for most *Proteus* species and all *Pseudomonas* species, nitrofurantoin is widely effective against coliforms. Resistance develops slowly, and so the drug is effective for long-term therapy. A polyneuropathy may develop if prolonged courses of therapy are used, especially in elderly patients. Unfortunately, effective urine levels may not be obtained if the glomerular filtration rate is significantly reduced, especially if the creatinine clearance is less than 80 milliliters per minute.

Sulfas Sulfas are effective against most gram-negative coliforms but not against *Pseudomonas* and *Proteus*.

Tetracycline This drug has only limited use because resistance develops rapidly. It should be used only occasionally, for short-term treatment. It is excreted primarily by the kidneys. If renal function is impaired, lower doses may be required to avoid liver toxicity. Tetracycline has an antianabolic activity, which may appear as a rising level of blood urea nitrogen when renal function is significantly impaired. Absorption may be impaired by milk, the divalent and trivalent cations in many antacids, and by a high stomach pH from the absorbable antacids. When renal failure is a problem, doxycycline, which is excreted primarily through the feces, may be used.

Miscellaneous Infections

Herpes simplex, the virus that causes fever blisters, on rare occasions causes severe pneumonia or meningitis. Such infections are serious and are more apt to occur in old people.

Fungal diseases, fairly rare generally, are seen chiefly in old people with defective immune systems.

PROBLEMS WITH ANTIBIOTICS

Incomplete intestinal absorption of such broad-spectrum antibiotics as ampicillin and tetracycline affects the flora of the large intestine, often resulting in the overgrowth of *Proteus, Pseudomonas,* staphylocci, and monilial organisms. This may lead to severe nausea, indigestion, abdominal pain, flatulence, diarrhea, and fecal incontinence. Dermatitis of the anus and vulva, with severe itching, may occur. This last problem may be prolonged and severe.

Because most antibiotics are excreted by the kidneys, the decline with age of renal plasma flow and glomerular filtration rate results in a higher and more prolonged blood level of many antibiotics, especially the aminoglycosides and the cephalosporins. This higher level is especially dangerous with the aminoglycosides, as they are nephrotoxic and ototoxic. Renal function should be evaluated by appropriate tests and the dose modified accordingly. When calculating the doses for these drugs, the standard formulas and nomograms involving renal function and age should be used. Prolonged blood levels have been noted after intramuscular injections of the procaine and benzathine salts of penicillin G. Sixty hours after an injection of procaine penicillin G, blood levels in those between ages 71 and 86 were four times that in young adults.

SUMMARY

We have touched upon the problems infections can cause in old people. As in the population generally, respiratory and urinary infections are the most prevalent infections in the old. The treatment of pneumonias in old people is generally the same as in the young. The approach is different in urinary infections, to a degree. These facts explain why we went into greater detail with urinary infections.

We now want to talk about anemia in old people.

Chapter 15

Vitamins, Minerals, and Hematinics

In the early years of this century it became evident that certain chemical substances, aside from the basic foodstuffs, were necessary for health. These compounds are called vitamins. They are essential in oxidation, reduction, and other complex chemical reactions that occur in living organisms. Vitamins enter such reactions but are not used up.

There is an enormous commerce in vitamins. Many people, encouraged by high-powered advertising, ascribe to vitamins some mystical ability to prevent illness, delay aging, and promote health. The fact is that water-soluble vitamins in excessive amounts are quickly excreted and probably do no harm, i.e., they may serve as expensive placebos. The fat-soluble vitamins A and D, however, can do much harm if taken in excess.

Many elderly people have capricious appetites, as we have pointed out before and a case can be made for supplemental vitamins. Technically speaking, such supplements are not drugs. However, when large doses of vitamins are taken, as by food fadists, for no apparent reason except to satisfy some morbid notion of treating nonexistent illness, then vitamins do become drugs, if nothing but placebos.

No group of drugs has been subjected to as much quackery as vitamins, minerals, and hematinics. Some manufacturers have made special claims for their own formulations. What might be a commonsensical approach?

People who are well and eat a diet containing meat, green vegetables, cereals, fruits, and dairy products do not need extra vitamins. However, those who are picky about their diet and dislike fruits and vegetables may need a vitamin and mineral supplement. What kind? A supplement giving all the recommended daily requirements of vitamins and minerals can be prescribed by a physician or bought over the counter. Such preparations may vary in price from about 6 to 35 cents per tablet or capsule. If one takes such a capsule daily for years, the price becomes a practical consideration.

Recommended daily requirements have been estimated by the Food and Nutrition Board, a group sponsored by the National Academy of Sciences and the National Research Council. Its recommendations are based upon the available evidence provided by experimental and clinical studies. The latest recommendations of the board are reproduced in Table 14-1.

VITAMIN DEFICIENCY

Causes

Vitamin deficiency occurs under three circumstances: (1) inadequate intake, (2) a disturbance in absorption, and (3) increased requirements.

Inadequate Intake   We have mentioned picky eaters who don't eat well-balanced diets. There are a number of people who, for religious or psychiatric reasons, don't eat a good diet. Strict vegetarians, who eat no foods of animal origin, are particularly prone to deficiencies of the fat-soluble vitamins. People who go on rigid diets for weight reduction may develop deficiencies. Many young people, who have an aversion to fruits and vegetables do not get adequate vitamins. In several studies, hospital patients have been found to eat an inadequate diet because of poor appetites for institutional food. Unfortunately, nursing-home patients may have poor appetites for food which may not be attractive. One cannot escape the conclusion that many Americans are simply pampered to the point that they can eat only certain foods prepared in special ways. This food prejudice of course puts an insuperable burden upon schools, hospitals, and nursing homes. Thus cold, unattractive food served in a perfunctory manner is an invitation to dietary deficiencies.

Disturbance in Absorption   Deficiencies in absorption occur in many illnesses. Among these illnesses are diseases of the digestive tract, infections causing diarrhea, and cancer in several forms. Ironically, several antibiotics may cause a persistent diarrhea in susceptible subjects, thus leading to deficiencies.

Table 14-1 Recommended Daily Dietary Allowances[a]

	Age, yr	Weight, kg	Height, cm	Energy, kcal[b]	Protein, g	Fat-soluble vitamins		Vitamin D IU	Vitamin E Activity IU[e]
						Vitamin Activity			
						RE[c]	IU		
Infants	0.0-0.5	6	60	kg × 117	kg × 2.2	420[d]	1400	400	4
	0.5-1.0	9	71	kg × 108	kg × 2.0	400	2000	400	5
Children	1-3	13	86	1300	23	400	2000	400	7
	4-6	20	110	1800	30	500	2500	400	9
	7-10	30	135	2400	36	700	3300	400	10
Males	11-14	44	158	2800	44	1000	5000	400	12
	15-18	61	172	3000	54	1000	5000	400	15
	19-22	67	172	3000	54	1000	5000	400	15
	23-50	70	172	2700	56	1000	5000		15
	51+	70	172	2400	56	1000	5000		15
Females	11-14	44	155	2400	44	800	4000	400	12
	15-18	54	162	2100	48	800	4000	400	12
	19-22	58	162	2100	46	800	4000	400	12
	23-50	58	162	2000	46	800	4000		12
	51+	58	162	1800	46	800	4000		12
Pregnant				+300	+30	1000	5000	400	15
Lactating				+500	+20	1200	6000	400	15

[a]The allowances are intended to provide for individual variations among most normal persons as they live in the United States under usual environmental stresses. Diets should be based on a variety of common foods in order to provide other nutrients for which human requirements have been less well defined.

[b]Kilojoules (kJ) = 4.2 × kcal.

[c]Retinol equivalents.

[d]Assumed to be all as retinol in milk during the first six months of life. All subsequent intakes are assumed to be half as retinol and half as β-carotene when calculated from international units. As retinol equivalents, three fourths are as retinol and one fourth as β-carotene.

Increased Requirements Under certain circumstances there is a greater requirement for certain vitamins. Among these is a preexisting vitamin deficiency that may itself cause diarrhea. To break the proverbial vicious circle, vitamins may be needed not only to maintain health but also to cure disease. Hyperthyroidism, fever from any source, and wasting disease from a number of causes, may all increase the need for vitamins.

Given the conditions, then, should all old people in hospitals and nursing homes be given supplemental vitamins? We don't believe they should. There are some very hardy eaters among the feeble old. Occasionally, we have encouraged people to eat better by stopping medication, including vitamins. On the other hand, we don't hesitate to prescribe vitamins when it seems likely that a deficiency is present or imminent.

Diagnosis

The symptoms of malnutrition, including deficiency states, may be subtle or confused with other diseases. What does one look for in assessing an old person

Water-soluble vitamins									Minerals			
Ascor-bic Acid, mg	Fola-cin[f] μg	Nia-cin[g] mg	Ribo-flavin, mg	Thia-min, mg	Vita-min B_6 mg	Vita-min B_{12}, μg	Cal-cium, mg	Phos-phorus, mg	Iodine, μg	Iron, mg	Mag-nesium, mg	Zinc, mg
35	50	5	0.4	0.3	0.3	0.3	360	240	35	10	60	3
35	50	8	0.6	0.5	0.4	0.3	540	400	45	15	70	5
40	100	9	0.8	0.7	0.6	1.0	800	800	60	15	150	10
40	200	12	1.1	0.9	0.9	1.5	800	800	80	10	200	10
40	300	16	1.2	1.2	1.2	2.0	800	800	110	10	250	10
45	400	18	1.5	1.4	1.6	3.0	1200	1200	130	18	350	15
45	400	20	1.8	1.5	2.0	3.0	1200	1200	150	18	400	15
45	400	20	1.8	1.5	2.0	3.0	800	800	140	10	350	15
45	400	18	1.6	1.4	2.0	3.0	800	800	130	10	350	15
45	400	16	1.5	1.2	2.0	3.0	800	800	110	10	350	15
45	400	16	1.3	1.2	1.6	3.0	1200	1200	115	18	300	15
45	400	14	1.4	1.1	2.0	3.0	1200	1200	115	18	300	15
45	400	14	1.4	1.1	2.0	3.0	800	800	100	18	300	15
45	400	13	1.2	1.0	2.0	3.0	800	800	100	18	300	15
45	400	12	1.1	1.0	2.0	3.0	800	800	80	10	300	15
60	800	+2	+0.3	+0.3	2.5	4.0	1200	1200	125	18+[h]	450	20
80	600	+4	+0.5	+0.3	2.5	4.0	1200	1200	150	18	450	25

Total vitamin E activity, estimated to be 80 percent as a-tocopherol and 20 percent other tocopherols.

[f]The folacin allowances refer to dietary sources as determined by Lactobacillus casei assay. Pure forms of folacin may be effective in doses less than one fourth of the recommended dietary allowance.

[g]Although allowances are expressed as niacin, it is recognized that on the average 1 mg of niacin is derived from each 60 mg of dietary tryptophan.

[h]This increased requirement cannot be met by ordinary diets; therefore, the use of supplemental iron is recommened.

Source: Modified from Food and Nutrition Board, National Research Council, 1974.

who may be malnourished? It is remarkable how quickly some old people will develop a slick, swollen, beefy-red tongue. If the person is confused, has diarrhea and dry scaly skin, it is likely that he or she has pellagra, a disease due to a deficiency of nicotinic acid.

The difficulty in diagnosis is compounded by the fact that a combination of deficiencies usually exists. For example, if in addition to having signs of the rarely seen classic pellagra, the patient is unable to flex benumbed feet and has heart failure, he or she also probably has a vitamin B_1, or thiamine, deficiency. The latter condition is called beriberi and is particularly apt to occur in alcoholics, who have a special need for thiamine. One writer, a physician, suggests that a great deal of misery could be prevented by enriching whiskey with thiamine, particularly when one considers that alcoholic dementia may be due, at least in part, to thiamine deficiency.

For some reason, riboflavin, or vitamin B_2, deficiency predisposes to skin infections and to cheilosis, i.e., soreness and ulceration at the corners of the mouth. Cheilosis is not always a symptom of vitamin deficiency, however, since it may be brought on by dental problems or simple drooping due to advanced age.

Vitamin C, ascorbic acid, is necessary for wound healing and the proper functioning of immune mechanisms. (See Chapter 14). In addition, it helps maintain the integrity of tiny blood vessels. A serious deficiency of vitamin C may cause scurvy, in which there is a marked tendency to bruise easily and to bleed from mucosal surfaces, especially the gums. Citrus fruits are especially rich in ascorbic acid. British sailors of another day were called "limeys" because limes were used on long voyages to prevent scurvy. Since many old people bruise easily, vitamin C deficiency should be kept in mind as a possible cause.

In recent years, a few scientists have recommended huge doses of vitamin C to prevent infections. The weight of evidence indicates, however, that there is no particular merit in taking huge doses because the excess is quickly excreted.

If one reads the fine print on the label of some vitamin preparations, he will see pantothenic acid, biotin, choline, inositol and para-aminobenzoic acid. Deficiencies of these vitamins rarely lead to clearly defined symptoms. In animals, there may be lethargy, convulsions, paralysis, skin eruptions, or gastrointestinal symptoms. Pyridoxine prevents a painful and disabling neuritis that occasionally occurs in patients who take isoniazid or hydralazine for a long time.

Choline is a precursor of acetylcholine, a very important neurotransmitter. In addition, it is lipotropic, having an important function in the metabolism of fat. At one time it was used to relieve the fatty deposition that occurs in some diseased livers. Later, it became evident that choline alone is ineffective in liver disease and that an adequate diet contains an optimum amount of this important but relatively expensive vitamin.

The need for inositol and para-aminobenzoic acid in human nutrition has not been clearly established.

Anemia

Perhaps the most serious vitamin and mineral deficiencies in a geriatric practice are those which cause anemia, a disorder in which there are too few or defective red blood cells. Vitamin preparations or minerals that are used to correct anemia are called hematinics. Hematinics, too, have been highly promoted for over-the-counter sale. Like other preparations, they occasionally are necessary, but just as often are used for a "tonic" or placebo effect.

When speaking of blood disorders in a book like this it is difficult to decide what to include. Hematology (the science of blood) is a broad subspecialty with a voluminous practice and literature of its own. It embraces sophisticated techniques and elaborate treatment. It touches on nearly all branches of medicine. In this chapter we shall emphasize blood conditions which we see frequently in a geriatrics practice and how they may differ, in detail, from the same conditions seen in younger patients.

Many drugs affect the blood-forming organs. We have mentioned a number of drugs that may depress the marrow, e.g., Butazolidin and chloramphenicol.

Other drugs, such as aspirin and coumadin, may enhance the bleeding tendency and cause loss of blood.

A number of nutrients are essential for normal blood production. Deficiencies of such nutrients are far more frequent in the old and, indeed, are rarely seen except in the old. Accordingly, much of this chapter deals with anemia due to nutritional deficiencies.

Deficiencies, of course, are caused by dietary inadequacies, poor absorption of essential nutrients or increased demand. Other than basic foodstuffs, the nutrients needed for blood formation are iron, copper, cobalt, vitamin B_{12}, folic acid, riboflavin, and pyridoxine.

For centuries, iron has been recognized as essential for healthy blood. Even today, much is made of the importance of iron. That iron is oversold, and overused by some people, does not gainsay that iron deficiency is a frequent cause of anemia. Iron-deficiency anemia may result from inadequate iron intake, from blood loss, or from poor absorption. Because of poor or capricious appetite, many old people simply don't eat. Iron is found mainly in liver, other red meats, cereals, and green vegetables. A person living largely on bread and milk products would be expected to become depleted of iron.

Chronic blood loss frequently depletes the body of iron. Bleeding hemorrhoids, oozing from the stomach or bowels, or bleeding from the vagina for any number of reasons all may cause iron-deficiency anemia.

If a person has too little hydrochloric acid in the stomach, iron absorption is impaired. Chronic nausea, vomiting, or diarrhea will also impair iron absorption. Once we saw Mrs. X., a patient with iron-deficiency anemia, for which the treatment was, obviously, iron. When her anemia failed to improve, it became obvious that she was losing more iron than she was absorbing from the iron tablets. She had been given the tablets regularly, but just as regularly she regurgitated them. Yes! Iron, in its various forms, is apt to be irritating to the gastrointestinal system.

Iron may cause heartburn, nausea, constipation, or diarrhea. It may, like digitalis, be responsible for loss of appetite. These symptoms are largely but not entirely confined to old people. Iron absorption is selective; the greater the need for iron, the more absorbed from a standard dose. Conversely, if a person takes more iron than she (usually) needs, much of it will not be absorbed.

Despite claims to the contrary, we have not been impressed that one form of iron is, regularly, less apt than another to cause unpleasant symptoms. If a pill causes nausea, a capsule might be tried. If both pill and capsule are upsetting, a liquid preparation might be tolerated more easily. In many instances, iron medication is not necessary, but, because iron is essential, many people want to be sure they get enough. Indeed, the risks of iron medication are not great, although indiscriminate iron use is coming into serious question.

If a person is markedly anemic and cannot take iron by mouth or cannot absorb it due to disease, iron may be given by intramuscular or intravenous injection. Such injections are not without danger: they may, on rare occasions, cause anaphylaxis, an abrupt, dangerous form of allergy. On the other hand, such injections may obviate the need for blood transfusion, which has serious dangers of its own. Iron injection is useful in diagnosis. It can replace depleted iron stores instantly. Then, if the anemia doesn't improve markedly over a period of weeks, the anemia was not due to iron deficiency in the first place, except in the case of continued bleeding. Admittedly, such diagnosis and treatment lack refinement. However, it may be preferable to elaborate clinical study over large distances in frail old people. We have used iron dextran (Imferon) injections on occasion with no serious ill effect. The injection may cause pain and a sore buttock as well as a stain on the skin if part of the solution leaks back about the needle wound.

Iron deficiency may be diagnosed by serum iron determinations and a study of the bone marrow, tests that are not always practical. There are times, however, when travel, hospitalization, and procedures are more disabling than the disease. Thus, regardless of scientific instincts, the physician, humbly and thoughtfully, must decide what is best for the patient.

In addition to iron, anemia may be caused by deficiencies of vitamin B_{12}, folic acid, copper, cobalt, pyridoxine, riboflavin, or protein. Anemias due to such deficiences may be stubborn and difficult to diagnose. They don't occur often as the sole result of a specific lack. Rather, they are more apt to occur in conjunction with general malnutrition or with other health problems such as cancer or infection. Many vitamin-mineral combinations contain these trace vitamins and minerals. Some contain liver extract, vitamin B_{12}, folic acid, and iron. Should one use them? Aside from being expensive and a nuisance to take, we do not recall seeing a patient harmed by taking vitamin-mineral supplements. A few people may develop heartburn or indigestion. It is possible that such medication could mask potentially serious disease such as the relatively rare folate deficiency. Our position is that we don't prescribe shotgun vitamins and minerals. We urge a truly well-balanced diet instead. On the other hand, if a person feels more secure taking them, we prescribe the most complete preparation for the money.

Generally, deficiencies of iron, cobalt, or copper cause a microcytic anemia, in which the red blood cells are smaller than normal. Deficiencies of vitamin B_{12} and folic acid, however, cause a macrocytic anemia, which is manifested by larger than normal red cells in the blood. People with microcytic anemia generally do not have a deficiency of white blood cells and platelets. With macrocytic anemia, though, there is apt to be a deficiency of white cells and platelets.

Vitamin B_{12} deficiency causes a condition called pernicious anemia, which is manifested by weakness, neuritis, and a tendency to develope infections. Folic acid deficiency is seen principally in people who have chronic diarrhea. These macrocytic anemias are rare compared to the anemia resulting from iron deficiency or blood loss.

Vitamins and mineral preparations have their detractors as well as their advocates. Such preparations have a decided placebo effect. Injections of vitamin preparations have long been used simply to assure a patient that something is being done. Rarely, it is possible that such treatment could mask serous illness. We deplore the use of such preparations if they are hastily prescribed without an attempt at understanding the patient's problem. On the other hand, we cannot deny that they are occasionally helpful, as placebos if not for their biochemical effects.

Other Vitamins and Minerals

So far we have considered the water-soluble vitamins and the minerals iron, cobalt, and copper. Certainly, calcium and phosphorus are necessary for normal healthy bones. There is a tendency, especially among elderly women, to lose these essential minerals and to develop osteoporosis. For reasons not fully understood, this bone-thinning tendency cannot always be prevented even when the diet is entirely adequate.

Among the factors affecting bone, though, is vitamin D, a fat-soluble vitamin that is usually stored in adequate supply in nearly all adults. A deficiency causes rickets in susceptible infants. Rickets results in malformed bones, as well as other abnormalities. In an effort to maintain normal bone through treatment with vitamin D, rare patients, some with medical approval, have taken large doses of vitamin D only to develop kidney stones, kidney failure, and other signs of hypercalcemia. In rare instances of hypocalcemia, vitamin D is used cautiously to maintain normal amounts of calcium in the blood.

Vitamin A, or carotene, is abundant in butter, cream, carrots, and other yellow vegetables. It is essential for a healthy skin and for the chemical processes that allow the retinae to react to visual stimuli. People who eat many carrots are apt to develop yellow skin, usually most obviously in the palms of the hands. At the same time the urine and blood serum will have an abnormal yellow color, reflecting carotenemia, a harmless but sometimes confusing condition.

Vitamin E was found essential to the development of normal rat embryos. On this bit of evidence and a great amount of publicity, it came to be called the fertility vitamin. Since fertility and libido are connected in the minds of many people, vitamin E has enjoyed commerical success as a rejuvenator and as an aphrodisiac. There is no solid evidence that vitamin E plays any part in human nutrition. A syndrome from vitamin E deficiency in humans has never been demonstrated.

Vitamin K is necessary for the normal clotting of blood. Unlike other vitamins, it can be manufactured in the digestive tract in the presence of bile salts and certain bacteria. Accordingly, a deficiency is seen principally in the newborn and in people who have an obstructed flow of bile, as occurs in a number of liver diseases. Vitamin K activity is suppressed by warfarin, leading to reduced blood coagulability. This, then, is the way this blood thinner works, as mentioned in Chapter 7.

In addition to minerals already mentioned, the body requires small amounts of trace elements, as noted in Table 14-1. There is incomplete knowledge of these trace elements. It is known that magnesium deficiency exists in most people with delirum tremens, i.e., alcoholic delirium, and magnesium can affect the outcome in this serious malady.

The next three chapters will be devoted to pharmacy practice.

Chapter 16

Pharmacy Procedure in a Retirement Community

Facilities for old people have names and definitions that vary from place to place and state to state. Among these names are extended-care facilities, nursing homes, skilled-nursing facilities, geriatric centers and hospitals, and simply homes. Such institutions have been criticized when the problem has been, essentially, a poor understanding of just what services they were supposed to render. There is no doubt, however, that unscrupulous operators have been convicted for inadequate care at exorbitant prices.

Among the abuses of old people, a dishonest commerce in drugs has perhaps been the most frequent. Out of these abuses has come stringent regulation by state and national authorites. In many instances, however, a definite model for pharmacy service has not emerged. In the hope that we may help some of our sister institutions, we include now the policies and procedures of the pharmacy service at the Methodist Retirement Home and its nursing home facility, the Joseph F. Coble Health Care Center, Durham, North Carolina.

INTRODUCTION

The policies and procedures of the pharmacy at the Methodist Retirement Home and Joseph F. Coble Health Care Center are designed to meet the needs of the institution, its members and patients, and the health care personnel serving the needs of these members and patients.

The procedures are as simple as possible. They are designed to assure good practice; adequate records; proper charging; ready review of drug therapy; good communications between nurse, pharmacist, and physician; and reliable drug distribution. The procedures are designed to work as efficiently as possible, consistent with current laws, regulations, documentation, and other problems inflicted by a multiplicity of regulatory agencies, third-party payers, and their minions.

The policies and procedures listed here are approved by the heads of pharmacy, nursing, medicine, and administration. They constitute the policies and procedures and regulations of the facility.

The pharmacist may make adjustments in procedures as the needs arise and after discussion with those affected by the changes. The changes will be reviewed at the next meeting of the Pharmacy Service Committee if warranted.

PHARMACY ORGANIZATION

Pharmacy services are provided by Donald A. Holloway, Pharm. D., R. Ph. The pharmacy has no regular hours, but the pharmacist is at the facility daily, Monday through Friday, and once on the weekend for whatever time is necessary to perform all pharmacy-related duties. The pharmacist is available for emergency call.

When the pharmacist is away, he arranges for adequate pharmacy coverage, informs Nursing and Administration of the change in coverage, and posts the name and phone number of the temporary pharmacist at the nursing stations.

The pharmacist is assisted by such technical help as is required to perform a variety of nonjudgmental technical tasks at the direction of the pharmacist.

Locations of pharmacy facilities are:

1 Domiciliary building, Methodist Retirement Home (MRH)
   a First floor—pharmacy storeroom
   b Second floor—old nurses' station—for storing nonlegend drugs and issuing prescriptions only
2 Health Care Center (HCC)
   a First floor pharamcy—for HCC and residents
   b First, second, and third floors—drug room at each nursing station
I The pharmacist selects a single source for each drug entity. This will be dispensed for all orders for that basic product regardless of the proprietary

name used by the physician. The physician may request that a specific brand be used.

Products are selected on the basis of known bioavailability, problems with that entity, especially as reported in the *A. Ph. A. Bioavailability Monographs*, reputation and product–recall history of the manufacturer, the critical nature of the drug, and the cost.

II Drugs brought into the HCC by newly admitted patients may be used for that patient after they have been identified and the physician has authorized their administration. Pharmacy will supply the drug as soon as possible.

III Samples—sample drugs are not used.

IV Sources

   A Wholesalers—location and use.

      1 Darby (Long Island)—some generics, nonlegend drugs, and large orders when prices are competitive.

      2 Duke University Pharmacy—immediate needs and items not commercially available.

      3 King (Raleigh)—all supplies, same-day delivery.

      4 O.M.B. (Wilson)—all supplies, next-day delivery.

      5 U.D.M. (California)—phone collect, noncommercially available unit-dose packages.

   B Direct purchases

1 Ayerst	**5** Parke-Davis	**9** Upjohn
2 Abbott	**6** Philips Roxane	**10** Wyeth
3 Merck, Sharpe & Dohme	**7** Roche	
4 Merrell	**8** Sandoz	

Inventory Review

A list of drugs ordered from each company is maintained (see Figure 16-1). On a regular basis, the technician prepares a photocopy of each inventory list, reviews stock levels of each drug, and orders the drugs from the company.

Current Cost File

A current drug cost file (see Figure 16-2) is maintained. The file lists the name, strength, manufacturer, and *Redbook* AWP per hundred bulk, per hundred unit dose, and where applicable, U.D.M. invoice cost per hundred. *Drug Topics* AWP updated prices are reviewed every 2 weeks and new prices are posted.

PHYSICIAN'S MEDICATION ORDERS AND PRESCRIPTIONS

All medication orders are written by the physician or the physician's associate on the physician's order form (Figure 16-3) in the patient's chart.

The order should include (1) date and hour written, (2) name and strength of the drug, (3) frequency of dosage (4) duration of therapy, and (5) signature of the physician or associate.

UD	ALDOMET	250 mg	100
BLK	ALDOMET	250 mg	100
UD	COGENTIN	1 mg	100
BLK	COGENTIN	1 mg	100
BLK	BENEMID	500 mg	100
UD	DIURIL	250 mg	100
UD	DIURIL	500 mg	100
BLK	DIURIL	250 mg	100
BLK	DIURIL	500 mg	100
UD	ELAVIL	10 mg	100
UD	ELAVIL	25 mg	100
UD	ELAVIL	50 mg	100
BLK	ELAVIL	10 mg	100
BLK	ELAVIL	25 mg	100
BLK	ELAVIL	50 mg	100
UD	INDOCIN	25 mg	100
UD	INDOCIN	50 mg	100
BLK	INDOCIN	25 mg	1000
BLK	INDOCIN	50 mg	1000
BLK	SINEMET	10/100	100
BLK	SINEMET	25/250	100
BLK	TRIAVIL	2/10	100

Figure 16-1 Inventory review, sample page.

Orders written by the physician's associate (P.A.) for drugs other than those on the Board of Medical Examiners approved list (Figure 16-4) are at the direction of the physician. The P.A. will be considered acting on the physician's orders, and these orders must be countersigned by the physician within 48 hours.

Drug orders which are phoned into the HCC may be received only by a nurse and must be countersigned by the physician within 48 hours. The nurse receiving the order records the order on the physician's order form in the patient's chart, the name of the physician, and the nurse's signature.

Telephone Orders for Residents

Telephoned drug orders for residents may be legally accepted only by an R.N., L.P.N., or pharmacist. The person accepting the order is responsible for placing the order on the resident's chart.

The chart is then sent to the pharmacy for handling.

Pharmacy will not accept any drug order not on the patient's chart, and will accept *only* the patient's chart. The pharmacist and pharmacy personnel will not enter any order on the chart unless received by the pharmacist.

Drug Name	Size or Strength	Manufac-turer	Price	UD Price	UDM Price
ADEFLOR	0.5 mg	Upjohn	3.74		
AFRIN NASAL SPRAY	15 mL	Schering	1.37		
ALDACTAZIDE		Searle	12.04	125.24/1000	
ALDOMET	250 mg	MS&D	7.88	8.11	
ALKERAN	2 mg	BW	10.40/C		
AMPICILLIN (AMCILL)	250 mg	P-D	11.27	11.27	
AMPICILLIN	500 mg	P-D	21.83	21.83	
AMPICILLIN	250 mg	PR	6.50		
AMPICILLIN	500 mg	PR	10.75		
ANTIVERT	12.5 mg	Roerig	6.07	6.89	
ARTANE	2 mg	Lederle	2.30	2.71/C	
ASPIRIN AND CODEINE	30 mg	P-D			
ATARAX	10 mg	Roerig	7.65		
ATARAX	25 mg	Roerig	11.21	12.38	

Figure 16-2 Drug cost file, sample page.

PHYSICIAN'S ORDERS

Family Name	First Name	Attending Physician	Room No.	Hosp. No.

Date Ordered	Date Discontinued	ORDERS

Figure 16-3 Physician's order form.

For the Writing of Prescriptions by Persons Approved To Prescribe Drugs under the Provisions of G.S. 90-18.1

No controlled substances (Schedule II, II-N, III, III—N, IV, V) defined by the Federal Controlled Substances Act may be prescribed.

No parenteral preparations (except insulin) may be prescribed.

Any pure form or combination of the following generic classes of drugs may be prescribed, unless the drug or class of drug is listed as excluded from the formulary. No drugs or classes of drugs that are excluded may be prescribed.

OTHER CRITERIA:

According to N.C. General Statute 90-18.1, written standing orders must be used.

Every prescription and every refill must be entered on the patient's chart. A refill can be authorized by telephone if the refill is entered on the patient's chart and countersigned by the physician within 72 hours.

Amount of drug can be no more than 100 dosage units or a 90 days supply, whichever is less.

ANTIHISTAMINES
Drugs excluded under this generic category:
  Promethazine

ANTI-INFECTIVE AGENTS
Drugs excluded under this generic category:
  Amebacides
    Carbarsone
    Diiodohydroxyquin
    Emetine
    Glycobiarsol
  Chloramphenicol
  Erythromycin Estolate
  Oxacillin
  Minocycline
  Pediatric Tetracycline
  Clindamycin
  Plasmodicides
  Amodiaquine
  Chloroquine
  Hydroxychloroquine
  Primaquine
  Pyrimethamine

ANTINEOPLASTIC AGENTS
All agents are excluded under this generic category.

BLOOD FORMATION AND COAGULATION
Drugs excluded under this generic category:
  Anticoagulants

CARDIOVASCULAR DRUGS

CENTRAL NERVOUS SYSTEM DRUGS
Drugs excluded under this generic category:
  Psychotherapeutic agents
  Antidepressants
  Tranquilizers
  Benactyzine
  Lithium
  Respiratory stimulants
  Cerebral stimulants
  Sedatives and hypnotics
  Pentazocine

DIAGNOSTIC AGENTS

ELECTROLYTIC, CALORIC, AND WATER-BALANCE ENZYMES

EXPECTORANTS AND COUGH PREPARATIONS

EAR, EYE, NOSE, AND THROAT PREPARATIONS
Drugs excluded under this generic category:
  Any preparation containing an excluded drug.

GASTROINTESTINAL DRUGS

HORMONES AND SYNTHETIC SUBSTITUTES
Drugs excluded under this generic category:
  Parathyroid hormones and synthetics
  Pituitary hormones and synthetics

OXYTOCICS
All agents are excluded under this generic category.

RADIOACTIVE AGENTS
All agents are excluded under this generic category.

SKIN AND MUCOUS MEMBRANE PREPARATIONS
Drugs excluded under this generic category:
  Any preparation containing an excluded drug.

Figure 16-4 Board of Medical Examiners' approved formulary.

If no R.N. or L.P.N. is available to accept the order at the unit, the order must be accepted by a nurse in the HCC who may then inform the unit of the order if unit personnel are to administer the drug.

A prescription is a written order or other order which is promptly reduced to writing and is issued by a practitioner licensed in North Carolina to administer or prescribe drugs in the course of professional practice. However, drug orders in a patient's chart are specifically exempted as prescriptions by North Carolina law.

Drug orders in the patient's chart are converted to prescriptions on an MRH-HCC prescription blank (Figure 16-5a). The lines along side the posted and filled prescription are the back of the prescription for filing refill data.

The bottom copy (Figure 16-5b) of the prescription blank is attached to the medication order renewal list (MORL, Figure 16-11). This sheet lists only current drugs and is used in the HCC to simplify monthly renewal orders.

On the first of the month, the pharmacy technician prepares a photocopy of each HCC patient's medication order renewal list. The pharmacist adds comments from the patient's chart reviews, and the copies are given to nursing personnel for them to add any data about diets, additional treatments, and comments. After the physician signs the MORL as having reviewed it, any necessary change orders are made in the patient's chart, and nursing files the review sheets.

Class II Controlled Drugs

C-II drugs must be ordered on a prescription with the physician's signature. Thus orders for C-II drugs in the patient's chart may not be filled legally. The physician must leave a signed prescription along with the order in the chart. If this is not done, the pharmacist will prepare a prescription for the physician's signature.

Other Drugs

Administration of nonlegend drugs initiated by the nurse must be entered on the physician's order sheet and sent to the pharmacy for handling. The physician should sign the order within 48 hours. Supplies may *not* be brought from the old nurses' station in the domiciliary building for this purpose.

The nurse may not initiate other drug therapy without standing orders and then only after entering the order on the physician's order sheet. It is illegal to use medications from one patient's drawers to administer to another patient.

Other

All orders and changes in orders should follow the last chart entry. Orders should not be squeezed in as an afterthought after the physician has signed orders. Changes should be entered as changes, and not by scratching out and rewriting an order after it has been processed by the pharmacy.

Federal law prohibits administering a controlled drug to anybody other than to whom the drug was dispensed pursuant to a valid order. When these drugs are placed in a patient's drawer, they are dispensed to that patient. Administering these drugs, even a single dose, to anybody else is a federal crime.

PRESCRIPTION FILE AND PROFILE

Patient ___BALLOR, WALLY___

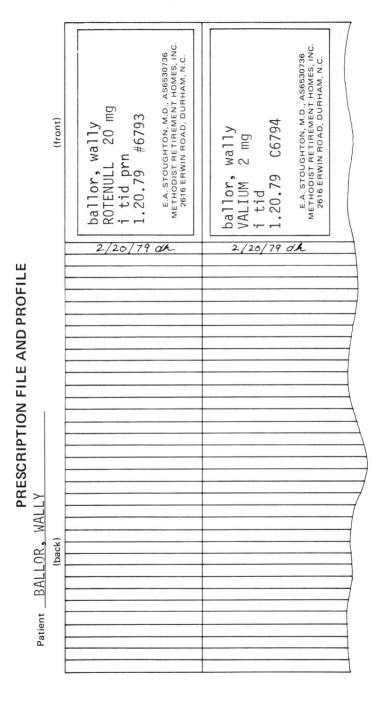

(front)

ballor, wally
ROTENULL   20 mg
i tid prn
1.20.79   #6793

E.A. STOUGHTON, M.D., AS6530736
METHODIST RETIREMENT HOMES, INC.
2616 ERWIN ROAD, DURHAM, N.C.

2/20/79 dh

ballor, wally
VALIUM   2 mg
i tid
1.20.79   C6794

E.A. STOUGHTON, M.D., AS6530736
METHODIST RETIREMENT HOMES, INC.
2616 ERWIN ROAD, DURHAM, N.C.

2/20/79 dh

(back)

Figure 16-5 (a) MRH-HCC prescription form.

155

```
ballor, wally
ROTENULL   20 mg
i tid prn
1.20.79   #6793
```

Figure 16-5
(b) Bottom copy of prescription form.

BASIC PROCEDURES–INPATIENTS

The following definitions are taken from conditions of participation for skilled nursing facilities:

Drug dispensing   An act entailing the interpretation of an order for a drug or biological and, pursuant to that order, the proper selection, measuring, labeling, packaging, and issuance of the drug or biological for a patient or for a service unit of the facility

Drug administration   An act in which a single dose of a prescribed drug or biological is given to a patient by an authorized person in accordance with all laws and regulations governing such acts. The complete act of administration entails removing an individual dose from a previously dispensed, properly labeled container, verifying it with the physician's orders, giving the individual dose to the proper patient, and promptly recording the time and dose given.

Standard labeling of drugs and biologicals   The labeling of drugs and biologicals is based on currently accepted professional principles and includes the appropriate accessory and cautionary instructions as well as the expiration date when applicable.

To meet these definitions and to ensure safe and efficient procedures, the medication ordering, dispensing, and administration routine is as follows:

1   The physician or physician's associate writes the order in the patient's chart.

2   The order is entered onto the medication record (Figure 16-6) by the nurse, or it may be left for the pharmacist to do later.

3   The chart is placed in the pharmacist's box.

4   Unless the physician orders the immediate administration of the first dose, the drug is not administered until the pharmacist has reviewed the drug order.

If the physician orders the immediate administration of the first dose, the nurse may enter the pharmacy and remove and administer that single dose.

5   The pharmacy technician reviews the order, assigns a prescription number to the order, prepares a prescription, enters the order onto the cart-filling Kardex, and places the drug in any carts in the pharmacy (see Figure 16-7).

MEDICATION RECORD

FOR THE MONTH OF _December_ 19 _79_

FAMILY NAME _Ballou, Wally_   FIRST

No. _____

ROOM _____

PHONE

ATTENDING PHYSICIAN

MEDICATION	HOUR GIVEN	1	2	3	4	5	6	7	8	9	10	11	12	13	14	15	16	17	18	19	20	21	22	23	24	25	26	27	28	29	30	31
Valium 2 g.	8																																
	12																																
	5																																
Retinil prn																																	

Figure 16-6 Medication record.

PHARMACY MEDICATION KARDEX

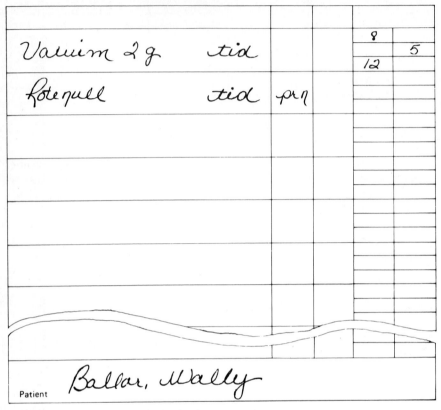

Figure 16-7 Pharmacy medication kardex.

6 The pharmacist reviews all new orders, checks the new drug against the patient's chart, reviews all procedures in **5** above, signs the order, and checks the medication record. Doses for the remainder of the day are placed in the patient's drawer and the new prescription and MORL tag are filed.

7 *Discontinued Orders.* Discontinued orders are forwarded to the pharmacy for recording on the cart-filling Kardex, removal from the MORL, and discontinuing on the prescription file. Doses in the system are removed by technician or pharmacist.

8 *Change Orders.* Change orders are forwarded to the pharmacy. They may be treated as new orders or they may be changed on the records as a change only.

9 *Emergencies.* When there is an emergency order for a drug which is not in the emergency kit or the pharmacy, the charge nurse will phone the pharmacist. When a pharmacy technician is on duty, the technician will phone the pharmacist.

Stop-order Policy

The following stop-order policies will be followed unless the physician specifies the duration of therapy:

1 Anticoagulants—5 days
2 Narcotics—5 days
3 Antibiotics—10 days
4 All other drugs—30 days

Drug-therapy Review

The pharmacist reviews all HCC drug therapy monthly and calls any potential problems to the attention of the physician on the MORL. Other problems may be called to the attention of the director of nursing or the administrator as the situation warrants.

The pharmacist checks for correlation among the pharmacy prescription file, master order renewal list, cart-filling Kardex, the physician's orders, adverse effects, and adherence to the physician's orders.

The reviewed chart is date-stamped and initialed.

Transfers Between the Domiciliary and Health Care Center

1 Entering the HCC. Patients entering the HCC will have all drug orders rewritten and approved by the physician.

Medications *currently* taken by the patient may be entered on the medication record by the nurse or pharmacist for administration pending approval by the physician.

2 Discharge from the HCC. Upon discharge from the HCC, all drug orders will be brought forward and filled by the pharmacist.

3 Return from hospital. All patients returning to the Home from hospitalization will have their drug orders rewritten.

4 Domiciliary Prescriptions. For eventual return to the domiciliary. A supply of plastic bags with a pharmacy label affixed and a 3 × 5 card inside is kept at the nursing stations on the second and third floor nursing stations. When a domiciliary resident is admitted to the HCC the nurse collects the prescribed drugs the patient brings, places them in the plastic bag, writes the names of the drugs on the card, and places the card in the file box. The bag of drugs is sent to the pharmacy. The pharmacist or technician checks the bag against the card and initials the card as being correct.

When the patient is to be discharged, the nurse pulls the card from the box and sends it to the pharmacy via the box. The pharmacist checks the card against the physician's discharge orders and returns those drugs which are to be continued. Drugs not sent to the pharmacy will be assumed to be in the patient's room and will not be filled and sent to the patient upon discharge.

For those patients who will be permanent residents in the HCC, the nurse will place the drugs in the bag along with a notation on the card that the drugs are no longer needed, and drugs, bag, and card will be sent to the pharmacy for destruction.

Drug Cart Preparation

The HCC drug distribution is a centralized unit-dose system. Individual patient drug drawers are prepared by the pharmacy technicians on the first floor of the HCC at the main pharmacy.

Drawers are filled from the drug-cart-filling Kardex:

    1 Drawers for floors one and two are divided into five sections. The first four sections correspond to the four administration times of the day and for prn orders for specific times. The fifth slot is for non-time-specific prn orders. The technician places a maximum of two doses of a prn drug unless only one daily dose is ordered.

    2 The drawers for the third floor are divided into four slots, corresponding to the four drug administration times of the day.

There is one drawer per patient per day. The technician prepares as many carts as possible, scheduling cart-filling days for maximum efficiency. The carts are tagged to indicate the day of the week they are to be used.

If unit-dose packaging is not available for a drug, a regular prescription container for the drug will be prepared, and this will be kept on the medication cart or will be transferred from drawer to drawer for each individual dose.

Drugs not available in unit dose packages from the manufacturer can be purchased on an interdepartmental requisition from the Department of Pharmacy, Duke University Medical Center or from a commercial unit-dose repackaging firm.

Carts are checked for accuracy by the pharmacist before delivery to the wards and the cart-check–sign-off sheet is dated and initialed for the dates checked (see Figure 16-8).

Controlled Drugs

C-II Drugs require a written prescription. The prescription is inserted in the Kardex and the technician records on the prescription the date and number of doses dispensed each day. When the drug is discontinued, the number of doses issued minus the number returned from the cart is subtracted from the perpetual inventory and the prescription is filed in the controlled drug file.

When filling the daily issue record for C-III to C-V drugs the technician also enters the figure twice, once for the number of doses *newly* issued for the day of administration and once for the number of doses removed from the cart on the previous day (see Figure 16-9). This allows the pharmacist to compare the

CART CHECK–SIGN-OFF SHEET

Month/Year

Carts for	Floor 1 day/by	Floor 2 day/by	Floor 3 day/by	Unit day/by
1				
2				
3				
4				
5				
6				
7				
8				
9				
10				
11				
12				
13				
14				

Month/Year

Carts for	Floor 1 day/by	Floor 2 day/by	Floor 3 day/by	Unit day/by
1				
2				
3				
4				
5				
6				
7				
8				
9				
10				
11				
12				
13				
14				

Figure 16-8 Cart check – sign-off sheet.

MEDICATION RECORD

FAMILY NAME / FIRST

Ballor, Wally

No. _____
ROOM _____

ATTENDING PHYSICIAN

FOR THE MONTH OF _____ 19___

PHONE

MEDICATION	HOUR GIVEN	1	2	3	4	5	6	7	8	9	10	11	12	13	14	15	16	17	18	19	20	21	22	23	24	25	26	27	28	29	30	31
December, 79 Dalmane 15 g	(1)	1	1	0	0	0	1	1	1	1	1	1	0	1	1	0	1	1	1	1	1	1	1	1	1	1	0	0	1	1	1	1
		1	1	1	1	1	1	0	1	1	1	0	1	1	1	1	1	1	1	1	0	0	1	1								
Valium 2 g	(2)	2	2	2	2	2	0	2	2	2	1	2	1	1	2	0	1	2	0	0	1	2	1	1	2	0	2	2	1			
		0	2	1	2	1	1	2	0	0	1	2	0	0	1	2	1	1	2	0	2	2	1									

Figure 16-9 Medication record. Notice that the figures are entered twice.

number of doses removed from the drawer with the number of doses recorded as administered.

Any significant problems will be called to the attention of the director of nursing, the administrator, or drug enforcement agency officials as the situation warrants.

These two forms constitute dispensing records for the pharmacy and are filed as such. The dispensing record for HCC patients may be used for as many months as possible.

When a drug is discontinued, the pharmacist or technician removes any unused doses from the patient's drawer and records the number of doses returned on the dispensing record.

Drug Administration

1   Only qualified nurses may administer drugs.

2   Medication administration scheduling is as listed in Table 16-1.

3   The medication nurse goes to each room with the drug cart, locates and identifies the patient, checks the medication record and doses in the cart, administers the drug, and charts the administration of each dose.

Doses administered to the patients at mealtime are given in the dining halls.

4   The nurse evaluates the patient's needs before administering a prn medication. Such medicines are not removed from their package until the nurse determines the need for the dose.

5   Medicines are not left at the patient's bedside unless this is specifically ordered by the physician.

6   *Errors*—medication errors are reported on a medication incident form (Figure 16-10). If necessary, the physician is informed immediately. The report is reviewed by the director of nursing, the physician, and the pharmacist.

7   Unneeded doses are left in the patient's drawer. They may not be removed for future use.

Table 16-1   Administration Times

Regimen	8:00 A.M.	Noon	4:00 P.M.	5:00 P.M.	8:00 P.M.
qd	X				
bid	X			X	
tid	X	X	X		
qid	X	X	X		X
q4h	X	X	X		X
ac	X	X	X		
hs					X
q6h	6 A.M.	X		6 P.M.	Midnight
q8h	X		X		Midnight

DRUG INCIDENT REPORT

Patient _____ Room _____ Date _____

Incident (cause and results)

REPORTED BY _____

How can this be prevented in the future?

Nurse   Physician   Pharmacist

Administrator's Comments

Figure 16-10   Drug incident report form.

Drug Administration Records

New drug orders may be placed on the medication record by the nurse. The pharmacist checks this entry or may enter the new order.

New medication records are rewritten monthly by pharmacy technicians from the cart-filling Kardex. The new medication record is reviewed for accuracy by the nurse on duty before the end of the month.

Old medication records are sent to the pharmacy for billing and are then returned to nursing for filing in the patients' records.

Master Order Renewal List (MORL)

An MORL is maintained for each patient and resident (see Figure 16-11). It lists only current drug orders. The pharmacy technician prepares a photocopy of the MORL on the first of the month, the pharmacist adds comments and observations derived from the earlier patient chart review, and leaves them at the HCC nursing stations for nursing input and physician review. Any changes in drug therapy are indicated in the patient's chart, and the chart is sent to the pharmacy for processing.

Storage of Drugs in the Drug Room

1 *The ward drug room.* These rooms are kept locked except when in immediate use. Medication carts are kept locked in these rooms.

The drug room on the second floor of the HCC is used to store a variety of topical semicosmetic supplies, mouthwashes, shaving supplies, and other items used for personal patient care. Other floors needing these supplies may obtain them here.

The pharmacy technician reviews stock in this room and orders more supplies as needed.

2 *Refrigeration.* Drugs requiring refrigeration are stored in the refrigerator of the ward drug room.

3 *External use items.* Items for external use, excepting ophthalmic, otic, and small volume semisolid topicals, are kept in a locked area away from internal preparations.

4 *Poisons.* Poisons or chemicals not used in treating illness are not stored in the drug cabinet or storerooms with medications.

5 *Nonlegend drugs.* Nonlegend drugs stored at the nursing stations of the unit may not be taken to the HCC. This practice has allowed nurses to initiate drug therapy without following the prescribed procedures of order entry and record keeping.

Emergency Drug Supply

The emergency drug box is kept in the drug room on the third floor nurses' station.

1 The drugs to be stocked in the emergency box are determined by the physician, pharmacist, and director of nursing. The contents of the kit are reviewed at 12-month intervals.

166

Figure 16-11 Master order renewal form (MORL).

Content of the form:

MEDICATION ORDER RENEWAL LIST

BALLOR, WALLY

Patient

Listed are current drug orders for this patient.   Physician should sign to indicate approval and that the drugs are to be continued.

```
ballor, wally
ROTENULL   20 mg
i tid prn
1.20.79  #6793
```

```
ballor, wally
VALIUM   2 mg
i tid
1.20.79   C6794
```

Physician

Date (pharmacy date stamp)

2   Access to the kit is limited to those authorized to receive orders and administer emergency drugs.

3   The contents of the kit are listed on the outside of the kit (see Figure 16-12).

4   The kit is sealed with a breakaway lock. The kit is expiration-dated for the earliest expiring product therein and is checked at least quarterly. The patency of the lock is checked daily by the pharmacist.

5   Drugs administered from the kit are charted on the patient's chart. These drugs are administered only on the orders of the physician. The orders should be placed in writing as soon as possible.

"Stat" Drug Needs

A key to the pharmacy is in a sealed coin envelope in the emergency box. If a drug is needed *after* regular pharmacy hours, the charge nurse may enter the pharmacy and take a *single* dose of a drug and leave a written record in the pharmacy of what was taken (see Figure 16-13). The key is replaced in the Emergency box.

Evidence of abuse of this will result in immediate discontinuance of the system.

A limited number of controlled drugs are left in the pharmacy (see signout sheet). It is illegal for *anybody* but the physician to order the administration of these drugs.

The pharmacy technician or pharmacist will place the key in a new sealed envelope and reseal the emergency box.

BASIC PROCEDURES–DOMICILIARY

Procedure

1   The physician writes the drug orders in the patient's chart.

2   The chart is placed in the pharmacist's box, which is later taken to the pharmacy.

3   Pharmacy personnel type a prescription tag and a prescription label; date-stamp the order; assign a number to the order by numbering the label, the order, the prescription blank, and the prescription log book; file the prescription; attach the under-tag to the MORL; and charge the prescription.

4   The pharmacist reviews the prescription.

Unless the physician specifies a number of doses or days of therapy, or the need for the medication is obviously limited, the drug will be considered to be for chronic use and the physician will not be contacted about refilling the prescription. See Figure 16-14 for label formats.

EMERGENCY DRUG KIT

Injections

AMPICILLIN 500 mg	4 Vials
AMINOPHYLLIN 500 mg	1 Amp.
ADRENALIN	10 Amp.
CALCIUM GLUCONATE	2 Amp.
CEFAZOLIN ½–1 g	4 Vials
CEPHALOTHIN ½–1 g	4 Vials
DEXTROSE 50% 50 mL	2 Vials
DIGOXIN 0.5 mg	2 Amp.
DILANTIN 250 mg	4 Amp.
DIPHENHYDRAMINE 50 mg	2 Syr.
FUROSEMINE 10 mg/mL 10 mL	2 Amp.
LIDOCAINE 2% (cardiac) IV 5mL	2 Syr.
PENICILLIN GK 5 M.U.	2 Vials
PHENERGAN 12½-25 mg	5 Amp.
QUINIDINE GLUCONATE	2 Vials
SODIUM BICARBONATE	2 Vials
SOLU CORTEF 100 mg	2 Vials
TALWIN	4 Amp.

Solid Orals

AMPICILLIN 250 mg	
CEPHALEXIN 250 mg	
DIGOXIN 0.25 mg	
ERYTHROMYCIN 250 mg.	
LASIX 40 mg	
TETRACYCLINE 250 mg	
PHENERGAN 12½ mg	

Supplies

Pharmacy key	1
J&J Rususitube	1
med. disposable	
Needles # 20, 1½"	4
Tourniquet	1
Alcohol wipes	5
Disposable syringes	
3 mL	2
10 mL	2
50 mL	1
Tubex holder	2
Dilantin syringes	2

For patient _____

Nurse opening emergency box _____

Date and time box opened _____

Box refilled and checked by pharmacist _____

Date and time _____

NURSES' PHARMACY SIGN-OUT SHEET: EMERGENCY

Drug & Strength			Manf.	Patient	Nurse	Date	Time
CHLORAL HYDRATE	500 mg	(5)					
DALMANE	15 mg	(5)					
LOMOTIL		(5)					
PHENOBARBITAL	15 mg	(5)					
PROPOXYPHENE	65 mg	(5)					
DARVON & ASPIRIN		(5)					
VALIUM	2 mg	(5)					
CODEINE TABLETS	30 mg	(2)					
MEPERIDINE TABS	50 mg	(5)					
MEPERIDINE TUBEX	100 mg	(2)					
PAREGORIC		(4)					
TERPIN HYD & CODEINE ELIXIR		(4)					
VALIUM INJECTION	10 mg	(2)					
OTHERS							

NURSE: This form must be completed in all sections when you remove any drug from the pharmacy. Noncompliance will be reported to the director of nursing and the administrator.

Place the container from which the dose was taken on top of this form.

PHARMACY PERSONNEL: Set out one copy daily.
File all completed copies after pharmacist checks it.
Keep all blanks in the main pharmacy.

Figure 16-13 Emergency sign-out sheet.

THE METHODIST RETIREMENT HOMES, INC.
2616 ERWIN ROAD, DURHAM, N.C. 383-2567
PHARMACY SERVICE AM-3198048
DONALD A. HOLLOWAY, PHARM. D.
E.A. STOUGHTON, M.D. AS6530736

BALLOR, WALLY 1.20.79
ROTENULL CAPSULES 20 mg
TAKE ONE CAPSULE THREE
TIMES DAILY AS NEEDED
FOR PAIN.
                    #6793

(a)

THE METHODIST RETIREMENT HOMES, INC.
2616 ERWIN ROAD, DURHAM, N.C. 383-2567
PHARMACY SERVICE AM-3198048
DONALD A. HOLLOWAY, PHARM. D.
E.A. STOUGHTON, M.D. AS6530736

BALLOR, WALLY
VALIUM TABLETS 2 mg
TAKE ONE TABLET THREE
TIMES DAILY FOR NERVES.

(b)

1.20.79 C6794   30 tabs
1   2   3   4   5

E.A. STOUGHTON, M.D. AS6530736
METHODIST RETIREMENT HOMES, INC. 383-2567
2616 ERWIN ROAD, DURHAM, N.C.

(c)

Figure 16-14 Label formats: (a) standard label and (b) controlled drug label. (c) Auxiliary tag for a refillable controlled drug.

Controlled Drugs

See Figure 16-14b for label format for controlled drugs. The auxiliary label on the back shows when the fifth refill is made or the 6-month limit is reached.

The pharmacist types a new prescription (Figure 16-15) which is sent to the physician to be signed. When the signed prescription is returned, it is filed until the prescription container is returned.

The old auxiliary label is removed and attached to the prescription for which it was prepared and which is in the patient's file. A new auxiliary label is prepared and attached to the back of the container. The prescription is signed and stapled to the patient's file. The prescription file is also stamped with the new prescription number. The controlled drug inventory book is posted for the new prescription.

Prescription Pickup and Refills

Domiciliary patients may leave prescriptions for refill at the nurses' station at the unit. Prescriptions left by 10:00 A.M. may be picked up by the residents that evening or between 9:30 A.M. and 10:00 A.M. the next day except Sundays.

New prescriptions for domiciliary residents may also be picked up here the evening of the day they are written.

If the patient is *not* capable of going to the unit, the physician should so indicate on the order and the pharmacist will deliver the medication to the patient's room or apartment.

If the pharmacist believes it necessary or critical, he will deliver the drug to the residents and instruct them in the use of the drug.

Refills

Routine   Requests for refills will not be checked with the physician unless:

1   The drug is for a limited condition or the physician has specified a certain duration of therapy.
2   There are legal limitations, as with controlled substances.
3   There is evidence of over- or underuse of the drug.

Refill Checks   For certain classes of drugs or for certain residents, at the request of the physician, the pharmacist will maintain a rotating file to assure that the patient is not underutilizing certain drugs. Refill data quickly indicates over-use of a drug, but underutilization is more difficult to determine.

Drugs suggested for this review are:

1   Cardiovasculars
2   Anticoagulants
3   Antihypertensives
4   Thyroid Preparations
5   Antidiabetics

GIVE FULL DIRECTIONS FOR USE

For: __BALLOR, WALLY_____ Age: _____ Date: _____
    (First Name)   (Initial)   (Last Name)

Address: __METHODIST RETIREMENT HOME_____
                    (Street)

City: __DURHAM, NORTH CAROLINA_____ No. _____

℞ VALIUM TABLETS   2 mg   g or mL
   sig? i tid

   CONTINUING: C6794 1.20.77
   REFILL? x 1   2   3   4   5

D.

S.

VALID FOR NARCOTICS OR CONTROLLED DRUGS

No. REFILLS ☐

Refill_____ Times or_____ months

LABEL NAME, STRENGTH, and   authorization is given for dispensing by
QUANTITY unless checked here ☐   nonproprietary name unless checked here ☐

Source &
Lot No. _____ Pharmacist _____ M.D.
                                    (Signature)

Date_____ Price_____ B.N.D. NO. _____

Figure 16-15   New controlled drug prescription.

Prescriptions from Outside Physicians

1   The prescription is given to the charge nurse, who records it in the patient's chart. He or she indicates on the prescription that it was charted, and places the prescription in the pharmacist's box.

2   The physician for the Home reviews the order on the next visit to the Home.

3   Prior to approval by the Home's physician, the pharmacist will *not* fill such a prescription when:

    a   It conflicts with another drug order. In this event the pharmacist will consult with the prescribing physician or the Home's physician as events dictate.

    b   There is a legal problem involving old or out-of-state prescriptions.

    c   There is doubt about the need, especially with old prescriptions. In this event the pharmacist will consult with the patient to determine the circumstances and with the patient's physician.

Refill Prescriptions from Another Pharmacy

We may not legally refill prescriptions from another pharmacy. If the need is critical for the patient's welfare, a 1–or 2–day's supply may be issued if the drug is stocked and until the resident can meet with the Home's physician. There is no charge for this, but the need must be critical, it may not be for any controlled drug, and the issuance will be at the pharmacist's discretion.

Review of Drug Therapy

Per Order When new drugs are ordered for a patient, the pharmacist reviews the other drug therapy for that patient and calls any potential problems to the attention of the physician on the pharmacy communication form.

Annual If there are no intervening problems, the pharmacist annually reviews the drug therapy for the domiciliary patients including refill history, puts this on a photocopy of the prescription file or the MORL, and sends this to the physician along with any pertinent suggestions or comments. This may be done during the patient's annual physical. A list of residents to be seen is sent to pharmacy, the technician prepares the photocopy, and the pharmacist reviews them and sends them to the physician. Any changes in drug therapy are made in the patient's chart, which is sent to pharmacy for processing.

Labeling

The pharmacist supervises all labeling of pharmaceuticals. Pharmaceuticals shall not be transferred from one container to another except by the pharmacist or, if by a technician, the containers will be left together until checked for accuracy by the pharmacist.

Patients Incapable of Self-Medication

A number of residents and patients in the unit are no longer capable of safe self-medication. The pharmacy prepares unit-dose cassettes for these patients in a manner similar to the HCC. Nursing personnel on the unit administer these drugs to the resident.

Critical Drug Check

The pharmacy maintains a review system for assuring patient compliance with certain critical drugs whose proper use is essential for health. These drugs are generally those involving the cardiovascular system, thyroid, antidiabetics, and any other regarded as essential by the pharmacist or physician.

1   Each such drug-patient combination is recorded on a medication card. The cards are filed in the 2-week slot appropriate for their return date.

2   When the bottle is returned, the card is removed, updated, and moved to the next 2-week slot.

3 When the 2-week period is past, the pharmacist removes any remaining cards and visits the residents to determine why they are not in compliance and to help them return to compliance.

4 If necessary, the physician will be advised of the difficulty and it may be necessary to have unit personnel administer these drugs.

NONLEGEND DRUGS

The Methodist Retirement Homes make common nonprescription drugs available to the domiciliary residents at no charge.

Because of the great variety and duplication of such drugs, the questionable value of many, the deleterious effects of others, the overpricing of most, and the limited space available for storing these drugs in the home, the selection must be limited.

Residents wanting drugs other than those supplied may purchase them elsewhere.

It is the responsibility of the pharmacist to select safe, reliable, and inexpensive medications for free, nonprescribed distribution to the residents in the domiciliary area.

Stock is limited to analgesics, laxatives, antacids, some topical medications, cough syrups and lozenges, decongestants, denture preparations, and bland or soothing ophthalmics.

The following are not stocked: vitamins, sedatives or nerve pills, bromides, prolonged-action dosage forms (except aspirin), and beauty or cosmetic aids.

The exact contents are in Figure 16-16.

The pharmacist will meet with members of the Home, singly or in groups, to explain the policy and the reasons for the selection of certain products. Although this can be done during regular visits to the Home, a prearranged meeting at a time convenient to the pharmacist is preferable.

Because many nonprescription drugs may interfere with some clinical chemistry tests, residents asking for these items at the infirmary nurses' station are asked to fill out a card listing nonprescribed drugs they regularly use. This form is kept for pharmacy review when reviewing other prescribed drugs when laboratory tests are ordered.

All drugs stocked in the nurses' station and the unit are stocked only in that area. The pharmacy technician regularly reviews supplies of these items from a master order list (Figure 16-16) and orders additional supplies as needed.

When they arrive, the technician checks them in and takes them all to the Domiciliary area.

Items stocked here *may not* be taken to the HCC.

A monthly record of all nonlegend drugs, whether for use in the HCC, or the domiciliary building, is maintained. The record is sent to the treasurer at the end of each month (Figure 16-17).

NON LEGEND DRUG STOCK LIST

Source	Item	Size
PR	ACETAMINOPHEN 650 mg	100
PR	DSS CAPS 100 mg	100
PR	DSS & C CAPS	100
PR	GUAIAFENESIN SYR	4 oz
PR	MOM Liq	4 oz
PR	MOM/CASCARA	4 oz
PR	KAOLIN-PECTIN	4 oz
Merrell	CEPACOL MWASH	5 oz
Merrell	CEPACOL LOZENGES	24's
	ASPIRIN, BAYER	100
	ASPIRIN, BAYER	225
	ASPIRIN, TIME REL.	125
	ABSORBINE JR.	
	A & D OINTMENT	
	ANUSOL CREAM	
	ANUSOL SUPP	
	BUFFERIN	100
	BUFFERIN	225
	BEN GAY GREASELESS	3 oz
	CALAMINE LOTION	4 oz (ltd)
	CAROID & BILE SALTS	100
	CORICIDIN	24
	CORICIDIN-D	24
	GELUSIL TABLETS	100
	LIQUIFILM TEARS	
	MAALOX TABLETS # 1	
	MAALOX SUSP	12–26 oz
	MENTHOLATUM	1oz
	MODANE TABLETS	100
	MILK OF MAGNESIA TABS	100
	MYLANTA SUSP	12 oz
	MINERAL OIL EXTRA HEAVY	12 oz
	NEOSPORIN OINT	1 oz
	NEOSYNEPHRINE ½%	DROPS SPRAY
	NIVEA OIL	4 oz
	NUPERCAINAL SUPP	12
	NUPERCAINAL OINT	1 oz

Figure 16-16 Nonlegend drug stock list, sample page.

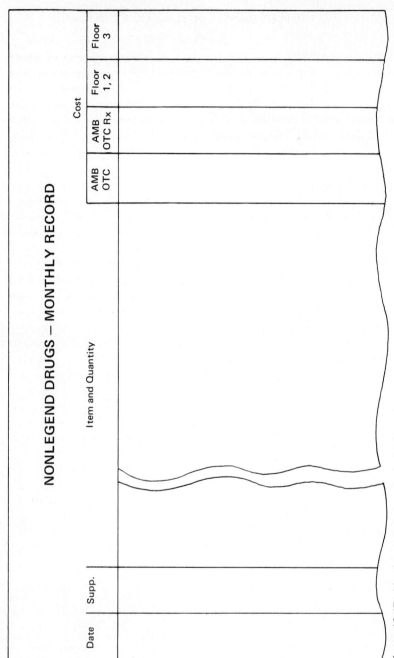

Figure 16-17 Monthly record of nonlegend drugs.

176

Single Doses of Nonprescription Drugs

A function of the resident assistants (R.A.s) and L.P.N.s at the nurses' station on the second floor of the domiciliary building has been the issuance of whole bottles of nonlegend drugs to the residents upon their request. These drugs have been selected by the pharmacist as being relatively safe and effective.

These personnel are authorized to administer single doses of these drugs upon the request of a resident when the resident does not wish a full container of the drug. However these nonprofessional personnel must not attempt to diagnose or prescribe a product nor to use another patient's medicines.

LABORATORY TESTS

Many drugs have been reported to interfere with various laboratory tests to a greater or lesser extent. Although there is reason to believe the extent is lesser, it is still desired to advise the physician when the possibility exists.

When results of laboratory tests are returned to the HCC, the pharmacist reviews the results for any abnormal values. If such abnormal values are found, the pharmacist reviews the patient's drug therapy and compares this with *Hansten's Drug Interactions*.

If there is a possiblity that the abnormality is due to the drug, the pharmacist prepares a *drug-clinical chemistry review form* (Figure 16-18) and returns the form to the physician's desk.

INSERVICE EDUCATION

The pharmacist prepares a series of taped discussions for inservice education. These tapes are in the possession of the director of nursing.

Tapes may be signed out by individual nurses to listen to at their own leisure.

OTHER PHARMACIST FUNCTIONS

The pharmacist serves on the following committees:

1 *Utilization review committee.* This meets once every 4 weeks to determine eligibility for Medicare.
2 *Pharmacy committee.* The pharmacist acts as secretary.
3 *Infection control committee.*
4 *Patient care committee.* Meets once weekly to review the care of selected patients.

DRUG–CLINICAL CHEMISTRY REVIEW FORM

Patient   Date

Laboratory Tests Ordered (to be filled in by nurse)

1.
2.
3.
4.
5.

Drug Therapy (drug, strength, and regimen) (by pharmacist)

1.
2.
3.
4.
5.
6.
7.
8.
9.
10.

The following interferences have been reported:

Figure 16-18   Drug – clinical chemistry review form.

PHARMACY TECHNICIAN

The pharmacy technician performs a variety of nonjudgmental tasks at the direction of the pharmacist:

1 Fills unit-dose drawers and all related tasks of preparing drawers, gathering empty cassettes, and maintaining records of controlled drugs issued in the drawers.
2 Fills and refills prescriptions and maintains appropriate charging and profile records.

No work done by the technician in **1** and **2** above will be released until approved by the pharmacist regardless of pressure by patient, nurse, or administrator. The physician may issue a drug on his or her own authority as one who is allowed to dispense.

3 Maintains current price information for most advantageous reimbursement by third–party payers.
5 Maintains cleanliness and order in the pharmacy.
6 Performs a variety of inventory control and purchasing functions. The technician checks and reviews stock levels in the pharmacies, second floor HCC drug room, and the nonlegend stock in the unit nurses' station, orders needed supplies from approved sources, checks them in, and places the supplies on the shelf. The technician also returns unneeded, outdated, and recalled items.
7 Prepares new medication records.
8 Prepares and maintains the master order list and prepares photocopies of this as needed for monthly HCC patient drug review.
9 The evening technician assists the pharmacist in all phases of preparing new drug orders for domiciliary and HCC patients and delivers drugs to the wards.

INSPECTIONS AND INSPECTORS

Pharmacy operations are susceptible to various state and federal inspections involving controlled drugs, Medicare, Medicaid, and the North Carolina Board of Pharmacy.

We are required to cooperate with these inspectors and they are required to come only during our normal business hours. The pharmacy is closed during the day while the technicians perform a variety of nonjudgmental tasks and is not officially open until the pharmacist arrives.

However the technicians may cooperate with these people despite their arrival at a nonbusiness hour.

PHARMACY CHARGING

Domiciliary Patients

1 *E. D. S.-covered patients* (N. C. welfare). A 30-day supply is issued and the program is charged Redbook AWP plus a fee of $2.50.

2 *Others*. Up to a 100-day supply is issued. The charge is Redbook AWP plus a fee of $2.50 per month supply.

Health Care Facility Patients

The number of doses administered is obtained from the previous month's medication record.

1 *E. D. S.-covered patients*. Same as for domiciliary patients.
2 *Others*. The patient is charged:
    A) Redbook AWP cost *plus*:
    B) An initial handling charge if the order originated that month *plus*:
    C) A fee per dose with a minimum monthly fee.

FORMS AND RECORDS TO BE POSTED

Pharmacy

Domiciliary prescription file book.
Health Care Center prescription file book.
Blue Cross/Blue Shield charge forms.
M. R. H. white sheet charge forms.
E. D. S. charge forms.

Nursing

Medication records.

Daily Charging System *(Residents and Individual Containers)*

1 *New Prescriptions*. File the prescription in the prescription file book and charge either BC/BS or E. D. S. plus the white sheet.

2 *Refills*. Indicate refill on the prescription record book and charge as above.

Monthly Charging and Refill Records—Health Care Center

1 Using the patient's medication record, record the number of doses administered over the month's period, date for the first of that month, and

2   Indicate the charge on either the BC/BS or E. D. S. sheet plus the white charge sheet.

FILLING PROCEDURES (REVIEW)

Domiciliary

1   Type the label.
Type the prescription.
Date-stamp the drug order.
Stamp the prescription number on the prescription in the prescription log book, prescription label, and on the drug order.
Attach the label to the container and cover with clear tape.
Place drug in the container
File the prescription in the patient's prescription file.
Attach the second tag to the patient's MORL.
Assign charges.
Take prescription container to the unit or the patient.
Record controlled drugs in the controlled drug record book.
2   If the order is for a refillable controlled drug,prepare an auxiliary tag as shown in Figure 16-14c, and stamp the prescription number on this auxiliary tag only.

Health Care Center

1   Type the prescription.
2   Type the label if necessary.
3   Date-stamp the order.
4   Stamp the prescription number on the prescription, the prescription log book, prescription label (if needed), and on the drug order.
5   Attach the label to the prescription label if necessary, and cover with clear adhesive tape.
6   Enter the new order on the cart-filling Kardex.
7   Place doses in drawers.
8   Pharmacist files the prescription in the patient's prescription file, attaches the second tag to the patient's MORL, checks all technician's work, and enters the order in the medication record.

Refill Prescriptions

1   Place drug into the bottle.
2   Record date and number of doses on auxiliary tag on container.
3   Record date and number of doses in patient's prescription file.
4   Assign charges.

5 Leave the filled container and used stock bottle for pharmacist to check.

6 If a controlled drug, subtract from the controlled drug record *and* if approaching the legal expiration of a controlled drug order, prepare a new prescription for the physician's signature.

7 Pharmacist checks all the technician's work.

REFERENCES

1 *Standards for Certification and Participation in Medicare and Medicaid Programs,* Reg. No. 39, USDHEW, 1974, pp. 2238–2257.

Chapter 17

The Pharmacist's Roles in the Nursing Home

The pharmacist serving an extended-care facility has the opportunity and obligation to assume a major role in the safe and rational utilization of drugs. The opportunites in such a facility are possibly even greater than they would be in many hospitals. There are several reasons for this. There is less tendency to be overwhelmed by conflicting interests, so often seen in large hospitals. Because of a different structure, the pharmacist is better able to define and refine functions and responsiblities with a minimum number of committees and meetings. Decisions often can be made on an informal basis with adminstrators, nurses, and physicians working together. This freedom can be a stimulus to exert one's best efforts. Physicians do not see patients in nursing homes as often to evaluate them as they do in hospitals. In many cases the physician may see the patient only at 30-day intervals, as required by Medicare regulations. Because of the slower pace, it is possible to use qualified pharmacy assistants extensively, thus minimizing the technical functions of the pharmacist. This division of labor allows the pharmacist to make more general decisions, review technicians' work, review and monitor drug therapy, and perform professional functions which cannot be delegated.

The pace of work for the nurse is also different. The nurse in the nursing home, while usually busy, is not generally under pressure. Thus it is possible for the pharmacist to spend some time chatting informally with the nurses about drugs, patients, and treatment plans. In extended-care facilities, there are fewer registered nurses and more licensed practical nurses. The latter tend to be less knowledgeable about drugs and to require more instruction about their use.

Medicare requires the pharmacist to perform monthly chart reviews and to monitor drug therapy. Physicians cannot order these reviews stopped, even if they want to do so. The exact functions of the pharmacist, and the extent to which they are performed are determined by the nature and quality of the physician and the nursing services, as well as by the pharmacist's own interests.

The general responsibilities of the pharmacist are in the areas of (1) administration, (2) distribution, (3) education, (4) clinical monitoring, and, possibly, (5) primary health care. This last function may be of value where medical attention is not always available or is merely perfunctory.

ADMINISTRATION

The general administrative responsibilities of a pharmacist include:

1   Preparing, maintaining, and enforcing written policies and procedures for the pharmacy.
2   Maintaining legal standards for all functions relating to the pharmacy.
3   Preparing required quarterly reports of pharmacy functions.
4   Selecting drug sources.
5   Supervising work and functions of pharmacy technicians.
6   Serving as secretary of the Pharmacy Committee.

DISTRIBUTION

The primary function and responsibility of the institutional pharmacist is to ensure a safe, efficient, and functional drug distribution system. Unless patients receive their drugs reliably and accurately, the efforts of the physician and of the pharmacist will be in vain. The policies and procedures described in Chapter 16 outline our pharmacy system. It has worked well for us. It helps us to keep up with drug orders, with the physician's monthly review, and with billing—all with no nurse involvement until the drug is to be administered. The system makes use of good technicians operating with minimal supervision. The only waste of the pharmacist's time is the legal requirement of checking drug drawers before the technician delivers them. After many months of checking, we find that conscientious technicans go months without making an error. The errors that they do make are noticed immediately by nurses when checking the drugs against the medication record. Our feelings are that with good technicians, drawer checking is unduly costly and time-consuming and adds nothing to patient safety.

EDUCATION

The pharmacist has an educational function. It is the pharmacist's duty to inform physicians, nurses, and others about drugs and pharmacy procedure. This educational function may range from formal lectures to informal discussions, consultations, and occasional chats—all with the purpose of relaying information about the safe and effective use of drugs. Any pharmacist who has tried to give a lecture to a group of nurses in a nursing home has probably found it difficult to assemble and hold any number of them. A suitable alternative is to tape-record talks on a variety of subjects and make the tapes available to the nurses via a sign-out system. This allows the nurses to take the tapes home and listen to them at their convenience and without interruption. Another less formal method is to go by the nursing station in the evenings to check for any pharmacy-related problems. These discussions can be helpful and pleasant for the pharmacist as well.

In most instances it is the patient who determines the success or failure of drug therapy. Thus success or failure may depend upon the person least knowledgeable about diseases, drugs, drug therapy, and drug administration. Unless this person performs properly, all the diagnostic and therapeutic skills of the physician, the research and manufacturing skills of the pharmaceutical industry, and the efforts of the pharmacist and other ancillary personnel will be wasted. The physician should inform the patient about the basics of his or her disease and treatment. The pharmacist should stress the need for proper use of the medicine, how the drug is to be taken, and precautions regarding side effects and the use of other prescribed or nonprescribed medicines. Patient education begins with the prescription label. Capital letters enable old eyes to read the label more easily. Complete sentences indicate how, when, and why the medicine is to be taken. For example:

TAKE 1 TABLET 4 TIMES DAILY BEFORE BREAKFAST, LUNCH, DINNER, AND AT BEDTIME FOR 10 DAYS UNTIL ALL ARE TAKEN. (FOR THE INFECTION).

or

TAKE 1 TABLET EVERY MORNING BEFORE BREAKFAST WITHOUT FAIL. (FOR THE HEART).

The pharmacist should reinforce the label by instructing the patient and answering any questions.

CLINICAL MONITORING AND REVIEWING

There are four ways of monitoring drugs. These include monitoring (1) drug therapy itself, (2) the patient's chart, (3) the drug profile (or administration record), and (4) the observations of the nursing staff and the patient.

The nurses are with the patients much of the time, see them function, know their problems, and are aware of changes in their condition. Unfortunately, not all the nurse's knowledge about the changing condition of the patient appears in the chart. When the patient is admitted to the extended-care facility, the chart should list all diagnoses and evaluations by the physician. In addition, the patient's medications should be clearly noted. The chart should present a fair picture of the patient's condition and treatment. Because the pharmacist receives the chart when any drug order is entered, and reviews it monthly as well, we do not have a pharmacy evaluation review form. Others have used such forms to outline the patient's illnesses and drug use. Our system combines the patient's drug file and profile into a single document which allows immediate review of the patient's drug therapy. When refilling prescriptions for ambulatory patients, overuse of a drug is immediately obvious. Another system is used to detect underutilization of drugs.

In the skilled nursing facility the patient's care is reviewed by a patient care committee. Nurses, a physician, a pharmacist, and other health workers serve on this committee. Of interest to the pharmacist are the comments made by nurses. These observations may never appear in the nurses' notes in the chart, but may indicate a drug-related problem. A patient who is feeling weaker, nauseated, and irritable may be overmedicated with digitoxin. Another patient with yellowing of the skin may be developing jaundice from Halotestin or chlorpromazine. When reviewing the patient's chart it is preferable to use the drug administration record for data about the patient's drug use and not the pharmacy profile. The profile may be a month behind actual drug usage. The drug administration record indicates what drugs are ordered, how they should be administered, and how they *are* administered—alas, *not* necessarily the same. The following points should be kept in mind when the pharmacist reviews the chart and drug administration record:

Is there an indication for the drug? Is the drug really needed? Is there a documented need for digoxin? Some estimates indicate that half the patients taking digoxin do not really need it. Is there a valid reason for using a major tranquilizer such as chlorpromazine? Of course, medical records are often deficient, but the pharmacist can help overcome this deficiency with repeated questions.

Is the drug appropriate for the diagnosis? If the patient is a little nervous or apprehensive, is a major tranquilizer like chlorpromazine justified? Is acetaminophen used for arthritic pain instead of aspirin?

Is there a better drug? And why is it a better drug? Or is it just a personal preference?

Is the dose appropriate? Digoxin is excreted only about half as fast in the aging body as in the younger. Diazepam and its metabolites are excreted more slowly and seem to have an exaggerated effect in older persons, so lower doses are appropriate. The patient's age is a factor used to calculate the dose of aminoglycoside antibiotics. Is aspirin or Indocin ordered as needed (prn) for arthritis pain and *not* given often enough to maintain a therapeutic blood level?

Will the drug do any good? Can glutamic acid hydrochloride (Acidulin) ordered for achlorhydria really make any difference, considering how many capsules are needed?

Are several drugs ordered for the same purpose? Are both diazepam and clorazepate ordered for mildly nervous people? Are similarly acting laxatives required for constipation, and are both aspirin and acetaminophen needed for mild pain or discomfort?

Is the drug having the desired effect? Has the patient responded as expected?

Are there any contraindications or problems with other illnesses? Is the patient with narrow-angle glaucoma being given an antihistamine for cold symptoms?

Are there any interacting drugs? Is aspirin being given to the arthritic patient who is being anticoagulated with warfarin? Is Maalox being given to wash down ampicillin or digoxin?

Are there any adverse effects from the drug? Do the nurses' notes or the social worker's evaluations mention nausea, lack of appetite, or irritability in the patient being given digoxin? Are there tremors, grimacing, tongue and mouth movements, or other extrapyramidal signs in the patient taking a phenothiazine? Is the formerly agitated patient now stupefied from tranquilizers? Is the skin rash due to ampicillin or the codeine in the cough medicine?

What monitoring is being done or should be done? How often are serum potassium levels performed on patients being treated with digoxin? Are blood pressures being taken on patients given antihypertensives or phenothiazines? Are liver function tests being done on patients given potentially hepatotoxic drugs?

Is the drug being administered as ordered? Many times drugs are not given as crdered. Although this is not too likely with such critical drugs as digoxin, antihypertensives, thyroid drugs, or antidiabetics, it is fairly common with the relatively minor drugs such as the benzodiazepines, analgesics, and laxatives. This is no cause for alarm. If the person does not need the drug—if there is no trouble sleeping and the patient is not particularly nervous and has no discomfort—there is no real reason to give the dose. It is usually more reasonable to have the physician change the order to correspond with the nurse's evaluation of the patient than to coerce the nurse into administering an unneeded drug. The other side of the coin is the regularly administered prn dose. Either the nurse is not evaluating the patient but is automatically giving the drug, or the patient does need the drug more than occasionaly. Either the nurse should be requested to evaluate the patient first or the order should be changed to reflect the actual needs of the patient.

Can anything be eliminated? Does the problem for which the drug was needed still exist? Does the patient still have the nausea for which the promethazine was ordered? Can the bisacodyl suppositories from an old bowel regimen be discontinued?

The comments and suggestions that occur during this review are written on the photocopies of the patient's drug record, which is prepared for the physician's monthly review. This allows the nurse to make comments before the physician makes the final decisions for that month.

Does pharmacy monitoring do any good? Probably.

Cheung and Kayne monitored 517 patients in three skilled nursing facilities for 11 months.[1] They claim to have prevented 70 drug interactions that could have resulted in hospitalizations costing a total of $40,000. They also claimed that monitoring helped reduce the average number of prescription drugs per patient from 5.9 to 4.6 leading to an annual savings of $25,000. Other studies arrive at different figures but with the same trend favoring this pharmacy function.

PRIMARY HEALTH CARE

A role for the pharmacist as a provider of primary health care has been advocated. This may be worthwhile when physicians are not available, or where simple advice is sought. Old-time pharmacists rendered good service in simpler days, but their role has changed. Among suggested functions for pharmacists in primary care are developing treatment plans and assessing physical status. We don't believe many pharmacists want to function as physicians or physician assistants.

REFERENCES

1   A. Cheung and R. Kayne, "An Application of Clinical Pharmacy Service in Extended Care Facilities," *California Pharmacist,* **23**: 22, 28, 43 (1975).

Chapter 18

Legal Responsibilities of the Pharmacist in Long-Term Care Facilities

The pharmacist providing services to a long-term care facility is faced by federal standards for skilled nursing facilities and intermediate care facilities under the Social Security Administration (Medicare) and Social and Rehabilitative Service (Medicaid). The effect of these regulations is to make the pharmacist generally responsible for all pharmacy services in the facility, and therefore a vital member of the health professions in the institution. The pharmacist cannot be only a "paper consultant" or a seller of drugs. Pharmacist and nursing service are jointly responsible for the ordering, storage, distribution, administration, and charting of all drugs.

Following are the definitions and requirements which are pertinent for pharmacies and skilled nursing facilities under Medicare.

Approved drugs and biologicals Those drugs which are included or approved by the United States Pharmacopeia, the National Formulary, the United States Homeopathic Pharmacopeia (these being the approved compendia of drug products), the AMA Drug Evaluations, or Accepted Dental Therapeutics, or those used during a patient's prior hospitalization, furnished to the patient with the approval of the hospital's formulary committee, and still required for the patient's treatment.

Controlled drugs   Those drugs which are subject to the Comprehensive Drug Abuse Prevention and Control Act of 1970. Common examples include narcotics, meprobamate, chloral hydrate, phenobarbital, Darvon, Valium, Librium, Placidyl, Dalmane, and Butisol Sodium.

Drug administration   The act of giving a *single* dose of a drug to a patient by an authorized person who is complying with all other laws and regulations which govern this act, including the *prompt recording of the time and dose* of the administration. Individual medication records are required, and unless a unit-dose is used, the person preparing the dose must also administer the dose. This last requirement assures that the person. administering the dose can also identify the drug. In the unit-dose system, the dose is labeled until the time of administration.

Drug dispensing   The interpretation of the order for a drug; the selection, measurement, labeling, packaging, and issuance of the drug for the patient or the service unit of the facility.

Pharmacist   An individual, licensed by the state to practice pharmacy, who has had training or experience in institutional pharmacy through residency programs, seminars, and related programs. The additional training and experience in institutional pharmacy should ensure that the pharmacist is aware of how his or her services mesh with other services in the care of the patient. So although not every licensed pharmacist is qualified to render service to skilled and intermediate nursing facilities, every pharmacist can prepare for such eligibility through various training programs.

Patient Care Policies

Written policies governing the nursing, medical, and related services are developed with the professional care staff, including nurses and physicians. Because the pharmacist must work closely with the medical and nursing staffs, pharmacy policies should be a *blend* of the requirements for the convenience and maintainance of the legal and ethical standards demanded of the nurse, physician, and pharmacist while meeting the requirements of the institution's administration. Among these policies and procedures must be the following.

1   An automatic stop-order policy—i.e., a policy that states that drugs will no longer be administered after a certain length of time unless the physician has specifically indicated the length of therapy. This type of policy usually specifically indicates stop times for narcotics, antibiotics, and anticoagulants.

2   Procedures for the storing of drugs and biologicals.

3   Provisions for an emergency kit, the contents of which have been approved by the pharmacy service committee.

4   A method for the nurse to obtain drugs from the pharmacy when the pharmacist is absent. The nurse may obtain only a single dose of a drug and must leave a written record of what has been taken from the pharmacy.

Pharmacy Services

The skilled nursing facility must provide a system for the distribution of drugs and biologicals for Medicare patients. The system must meet both accepted professional standards and federal, state, and local laws. This requires a pharmacist as defined above, who is responsible for developing and supervising *all* pharmaceutical services. Although not required to be a full-time employee, the pharmacist must devote enough time to the institution to perform all required duties.

What are these required duties in addition to those already listed? They may be divided into the following categories with some overlapping or duplication among these categories.

Patient Review Functions

1   The *drug regimen* of each patient must be reviewed at least monthly by the pharmacist, who reports irregularities to the medical director and the administrator. The purpose is to reduce drug interactions, duplications, unneeded drugs, errors in administration, and misuse and abuse of drugs.

2   As a member of the *patient care committee* the pharmacist meets and works with nurses, physicians, physician associates, physical therapists, social and rehabilitation workers, and dietitians in reviewing the patient's total care and in preparing team recommendations for individual patient care.

3   *The utilization review committee*, which must be composed of at least two physicians and optionally of other health care members and administrators, reviews medical care evaluation studies which identify the patterns of care in the institution and review extended care cases to ensure their efficiency, appropriateness, and cost effectiveness.

Committee Responsibilities

1   *Patient care committee* (discussed above).

2   *Utilization review committee* (discussed above).

3   *The pharmacy committee* is composed of at least the pharmacist, the director of nursing, an administrator, and one physician. The purpose of the committee is to oversee the pharmacy service and make suggestions and monitor the service for overall quality. The committee, which must meet at least quarterly, documents its activities, findings, and recommendations.

Although this committee will develop the policies and procedures for the pharmacy, the pharmacist must be familiar enough with the institution and its needs and with institutional pharmacy practice to act authoritatively in guiding the development of these policies and procedures and not allow others to make these decisions for or without the pharmacist. As a profession, pharmacy has come a long way as medical and social interactions have become more complex.

4 *The infection control committee* is composed of members of the medical, nursing, pharmacy, housekeeping, kitchen, and administrative staff. This committee establishes policies and procedures for investigating, controlling, and preventing infections in the facility and monitors staff performance. The pharmacist should have an understanding of sanitation procedures, disinfection, sterilization, isolation procedures, and mechanisms of the spread of infections.

Drug Labeling

The pharmacist is responsible for all labeling of drugs and biologicals, including any accessory and cautionary instructions and expiration dates. This labeling is based on currently accepted professional standards. This means that *nobody* else may label drugs and biologicals except the pharmacist or pharmacy personnel working under the direct supervision of the pharmacist.

Drug Control

The procedures developed for drug control should control and account for all drugs and biologicals distributed throughout the facility. Only those drugs which have been approved are used and they must be dispensed according to state and federal laws.

Records of the receipt and disposition of controlled drugs must be maintained in enough detail to enable an accurate reconciliation. The pharmacist must determine that drug records are in order and all controlled drugs are accounted for.

While the law does not state what system must be used, the pharmacist must make the system as "tight" as possible to prevent what is euphemistically referred to as "stock shrinkage." Before instituting a very complex system of records and controls, the pharmacist should remember that the function of a nurse is to provide nursing care, not to maintain voluminous records, and that the pharmacist has more vital functions to perform than to become obsessed by intricate records. However, if a relatively simple system indicates losses that cannot be explained by an occasional dropped dose, more complex records and accounting are needed.

A photocopy of the administration record listing controlled drugs may indicate what was *administered* but does not necessarily indicate what was *dispensed* from the pharmacy. So issue records are necessary even with a unit-dose system.

Reports

The pharmacist must submit, at least quarterly, a written report to the administrator and the pharmacy service committee on the status of the pharmacy service, staff performance, and related functions.

Staff Development and Training

The standards mandate an ongoing educational program for developing and improving the skills of the personnel, including training related to the problems of the aged, ill, and disabled. Records are to be maintained indicating the content of, and attendance at, such programs. Although the standard does not specify pharmacy involvement, it is hoped that the pharmacist contributes to this program.

The pharmacist can prepare talks to deliver personally to the staff, but because of the difficulty in getting a significant number of people away from duties to attend these talks, alternatives could include preparing taped talks to enable the staff to listen to the material at their convenience.

Medicaid Laws

The Medicaid laws place less demanding responsibilities upon the pharmacist. A pharmacist is required for consultation on proper ordering, storing, administering, disposal, and record keeping of drugs and biologicals. Automatic stop orders are required unless the physician specifies the duration of therapy. Self-administration of drugs is allowed only with the consent of the attending physician.

Unlike regulations for skilled nursing facilities which require the pharmacist to review the patient's drug therapy every month, intermediate care facilities require a nurse to review medications monthly and a physician to review them quarterly.

In addition to these federal laws, other legal considerations should be kept in mind. The purpose of this section is not to review all state pharmacy laws. These laws vary, often subtly, and what is legal, commendable, and progressive in one state may be just plain illegal in another. The pharmacist should pay particular attention to the following items and understand exactly the wording of a particular state's laws.

Prescriptions

Are drug orders in the patient's chart really prescriptions? Virginia law defines a prescription as an order for a drug transmitted from a legally authorized practitioner to a pharmacist. California law considers orders on hospital or emergency room charts as prescriptions. In contrast, North Carolina law indicates that prescriptions do *not* include drug orders entered on charts or medical records. North Carolina law also defines "hospital pharmacy" as a pharmacy as, among other things, a pharmacy in nursing and rest homes.

Drug Enforcement Administration regulations define a prescription as an order for medication dispensed to or for an ultimate user, not an order for medication dispensed for immediate administration to the ultimate user. Thus drug orders for hospitalized patients are not prescriptions.

The general desire of physicians in these settings is to write all orders, including drug orders, in the patient's chart and not rewrite the drug order on a prescription blank. Complicating this for the pharmacist using chart orders as prescriptions in a nursing or retirement home with an associated clinic is the general requirement that prescriptions be filed in the pharmacy and refills be indicated on the back of the prescription.

A simple method for handling this problem while maintaining a patient drug profile is discussed elsewhere in the section on the policies and procedures for the Methodist Retirement Home–Joseph F. Coble Health Care Center, Chapter 16.

Technicians

The legal limitations of technicians vary from state to state as the laws define the exact role of the pharmacist and what the pharmacist must personally do, as opposed to what the pharmacist may delegate to others and supervise. The pharmacist who is unwilling to become mired in the vital but purely manipulative minutiae of the operation of an institution and wishes to use technicians should become familiar with the exact wording of his or her state's pharmacy laws when outlining the duties of the technical staff.

For example, dispensing and compounding are different functions in North Carolina. Dispensing is the delivery of a drug to the ultimate user or a person acting on the user's behalf, while compounding is the combining of two or more substances into a single preparation. Colorado defines compounding to include the interpretation of the physician's order and preparation of the label and restricts this to the pharmacist. This greatly restricts the use of technicians in this area.

Ideally, with good technical assistance the pharmacist should have only to review the completed manipulative tasks of the technicians to ensure their accuracy and should then be able to concentrate on those functions which only a pharmacist can perform.

A properly qualified technician in North Carolina may work without immediate supervision while performing the various clerical, repackaging, and distributive functions in connection with a unit-dose system. However, the pharmacist is responsible for checking all such work before it can leave the pharmacy.

Emergency Drug Kits

There are various restrictions on the contents of an emergency kit, especially in regard to controlled drugs, the frequency of review of the kit's contents, who may have access to it and under what circumstances, who may accept orders to use it, and how it must be sealed.

Summary

Although there are numerous other pharmacy laws, those presented in this chapter cover the principal ones unique to pharmacy in skilled and intermediate care facilities.

Chapter 19

Summary

We have related our experience in the medication of old people. In doing so we may have been too technical for some and not technical enough for others. We have tried to appeal to those whose scientific training is limited. At the same time we have made an effort to bring up-to-date information to those who are conversant with recent developments in medicine and pharmacology. Our task has not been easy.

We have not tried to be all-inclusive. We are aware that we have omitted discussion of certain drugs that might have been included. We did not wish, however, to include a great deal of information above and beyond our own practical experience.

We have relied heavily on standard texts in pharmacology. Our book is based on the fact that standard texts do not give adequate treatment to techniques of prescribing for and treating elderly people. Our professional colleagues are often not as conversant as they should be about drug problems that we see every day. Accordingly, our book has attempted not only to instruct but also to raise the level of awareness in those who treat old people.

We have presented no new information, scientifically speaking. On the other hand, our experience may be profitable for those whose dealings with old people have been more limited than our own.

There are changes that occur with aging. We have tried to emphasize these changes as we went along. There are differences in absorption, utilization, and excretion of many drugs. We have mentioned volume distribution and drug interactions. We have spoken of nutrition and of vitamins, minerals, and hematinics. We have written of pain relief and cathartics, of drugs for heart and mind, and of placebos and placebo effects.

Since we believe neurotransmitter chemistry will assume an increasingly important place in medical research, we spent a good bit of time with neurotransmitters, particularly as applied to mind and movement. Indeed, we might have gone into greater detail, but we have kept our writing largely within the realm of our practical experience.

We had to avoid the tendency to become another textbook of medicine. For example, we left out a chapter on jaundice, by all means a worthy topic, but this is treated adequately elsewhere. In essence, we have included that which we believe most needs to be said concerning day-in–day-out drug treatment of old people.

How well we have succeeded depends, of course, upon the use to which this book is put. We shall be flattered if a few of our colleagues find it useful in instructing students. If one or more chapters become basic references for medical lectures we shall be honored. Short of plagiarism, we hope this book finds wide application.

For social workers and others for whom the field of pharmacy is only of collateral interest, we hope we have put together a useful volume. Often lay people can render great service to patients by an apt question to a physician. We hope we have stimulated some of these apt questions.

Finally, we may not have a book at all in the sense of a beginning and an end. It may be only a compendium of experience to which each reader may add or subtract. We shall not judge. We only hope that our readers will find it of some interest and some use.

Index

Index

74099